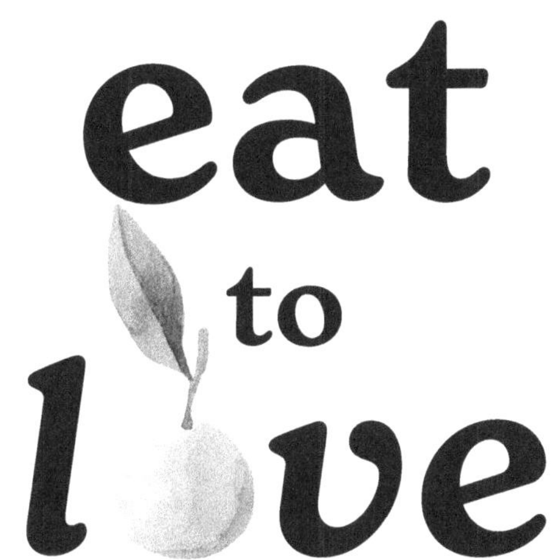

eat to love

Companion Workbook

eat to love

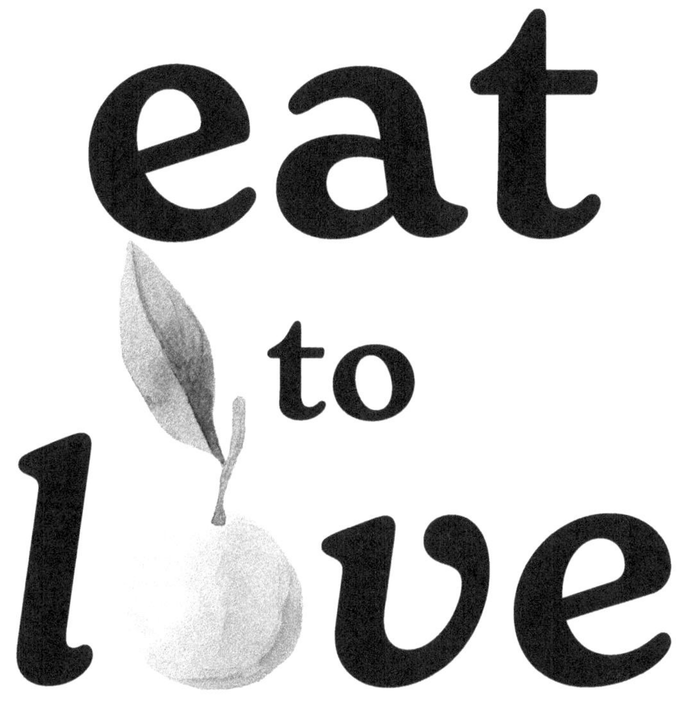

Companion Workbook

JENNA HOLLENSTEIN MS, RDN

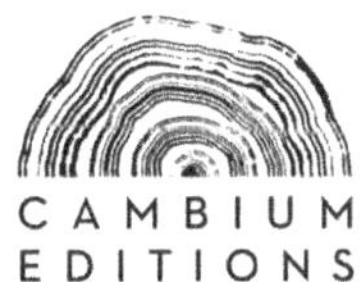

CAMBIUM EDITIONS

This book is not intended as a substitute for the medical advice of a physical or mental healthcare professional. The reader should regularly consult their healthcare practitioner in matters relating to their physical or mental health and particularly with respect to any symptoms that may require diagnosis or medical attention.

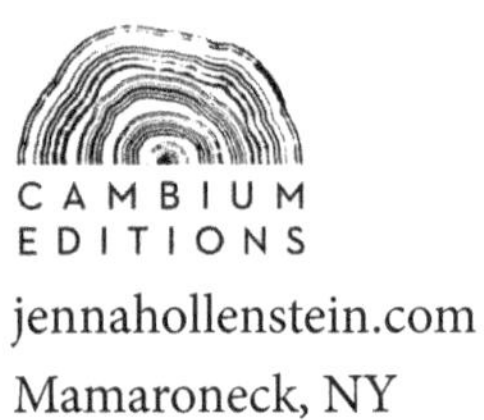

CAMBIUM
EDITIONS

jennahollenstein.com
Mamaroneck, NY

Paperback ISBN: 979-8-9945009-0-3

Cover and text design by Alex Hennig
Editing by Rebecca Beardsall
Proofreading by Dania Sheldon
Back cover illustration Georgina Luck

Introduction / 1

The Soil: Foundational Needs / 9

The Sun: Cognitive Shifts / 41

The Rain: Emotional Nourishment / 67

The Trunk: Satisfaction / 101

The Branches: Expansion / 117

The Air: Trauma-Informed Mindfulness / 149

A Final Word / 163

Additional Worksheets / 165

Introduction

Since *Eat to Love: A Mindful Guide to Transforming Your Relationship with Food, Body, and Life* was released in 2019, so much has unfolded—personally, culturally, and globally. We've lived through a pandemic that not only distanced us physically but also reminded us how profoundly interconnected we are. We've witnessed social and political upheaval, as polarization tears through relationships and the struggle for basic human rights grows ever more urgent. Meanwhile, the diet industry continues to thrive, with weight loss drugs entering the market, promising quick fixes, and fueling the never-ending cycle of self-criticism and disconnection.

On a personal note, I've also experienced deep transformation. My family and I left the city, finding new roots in the suburbs. I've crossed the milestone of turning 50, while my son just turned 10. My health has been an ongoing challenge, with chronic nerve pain, fluctuating moods, and what I suspect may be some neurodivergence—now intertwined with the complexities of perimenopause. Amidst these changes, I find myself often reflecting on cycles—how I am moving through the world at this specific moment in time, and how this influences my sense of self. These middle-aged moments bring me closer to the rhythms of life—where things are always in flux, always evolving.

Through it all, I remain deeply committed to meditation, Buddhist philosophy, and alleviating suffering in the world. I know in my own body how essential a peaceful, nourishing, and satisfying relationship with food and body is to that work. This workbook is an offering of the same companionship I've shared with my clients, now crafted to support you on your own Intuitive Eating journey. Perhaps some of what you gain from this work will compel you to also make the world a more compassionate, loving place.

What Is Intuitive Eating?

At its core, Intuitive Eating is about returning to your body's natural wisdom. It's an approach to food that rejects diet culture, honors your internal cues of hunger and fullness, and allows for the joy of eating without guilt or shame. But more than that, it's a healing process—a way to repair the trust that diet culture, societal pressures, and past experiences may have broken. It's about relearning how to nourish yourself physically, mentally, and emotionally.

This journey is not about perfection. It's not about following a new set of rules. It's about curiosity, self-compassion, and the willingness to unlearn and rediscover. Intuitive Eating isn't just about food—and it's not only about your relationship with yourself. It's about creating the conditions for your truest self to emerge. When you make peace with food, respect your body, and tend to your heart and soul in the ways they're quietly longing for, something powerful happens: you begin to show up more fully, more clearly, more compassionately. And that version of you—the grounded, authentic you—is exactly what this world needs. By doing this work, you're not only healing yourself; you're contributing to a kinder, more connected world.

What You Can Expect from This Workbook

This workbook is designed to guide you through Intuitive Eating in a mindful, compassionate, and realistic way. Because progress is not linear, I've created a visual framework—the image of a living tree—to help you understand how different aspects of Intuitive Eating relate to one another. This ecosystem model can help you determine, whether today or ten years from now, where your energy and attention might best be directed.

The Intuitive Eating Ecosystem represents the ongoing, organic nature of this practice. It's composed of several interconnected spheres that work together to nourish growth:

The Soil: Foundational Needs

This is where your journey begins. Without enough sleep, food, safety, and regulation of your nervous system, nothing else can take root. The soil represents your most basic creaturely needs—the conditions that allow you to germinate and grow into a deeper understanding of yourself.

The Sun: Cognitive Shifts

This is the light that supports your inner transformation. Here, you begin to soften rigid thinking, challenge the food police, and unlearn the diet mentality. The sun shines through nuance and complexity, helping you think differently, with more flexibility, compassion, and truth.

The Rain: Emotional Nourishment

This is the water that soaks into the roots of your heart. It's the ongoing work of tending to your inner voice—learning to speak to yourself with warmth, honoring your vulnerability, and creating space for your feelings without judgment. This is the realm of self-compassion and emotional bravery.

The Trunk: Satisfaction

With your foundational needs met, you can begin to connect with the experience of *enough*. The trunk of the tree represents satisfaction: enough chocolate, enough pleasure, enough quiet, enough nature, enough connection. When you are satisfied, you are free. You can return to your life without fixation, shame, or regret.

The Branches: Expansion

When peace with food is established, you naturally branch out into more advanced elements of Intuitive Eating, including stopping when comfortably full, engaging in regular and joyful movement,* and integrating gentle nutrition based on what your body truly needs. These branches don't represent rules—they are expressions of trust, connection, and care. They are what grow when you nurture the whole tree.

The Air: Trauma-Informed Mindfulness

Air is the spaciousness of presence. It reminds us to work gently with our nervous systems, to engage mindfully with life as it unfolds. Mindfulness might look like meditation, breathwork, a body scan, or a simple check-in. The key is discernment: learning to sense when to lean into discomfort—and when to step back and return later. This is the practice of honoring your window of tolerance.

Each of these chapters will invite you to reflect, explore, and practice:

- **Exercises for Journaling and Reflection:** Thought-provoking questions to deepen your awareness and reconnect with your body's wisdom.
- **Practical Tools:** Strategies to help you navigate everyday eating experiences with confidence.
- **Real-World Considerations:** Addressing challenges like food insecurity, medical conditions, and emotional eating.
- **Self-Compassion Practices:** Because healing your relationship with food is about more than what's on your plate—it's about how you speak to yourself along the way.

---

* You might notice that joyful movement appears here, in the expansion phase, rather than in the soil where foundational needs live. That's intentional. Movement is, indeed, a basic human need—we are born to move, and doing so helps us feel grounded, present, and alive. But for many of us, movement has been entangled with the diet mentality: something we do to earn our food, to shrink our bodies, or to punish ourselves for simply existing in them.

Reclaiming movement—on your own terms—often requires healing first. It asks you to disentangle movement from shame, pressure, and performance, and to rediscover it as something that connects you to joy, vitality, and embodiment. You don't have to be athletic. You don't have to perform. You just have to listen.

When movement becomes an expression of care, curiosity, and freedom—not control—it can once again become part of the soil and the branches. Something that both grounds and expands you.

Where Do the Six Paramitas Fit In?

In the original book *Eat to Love*, I framed the practice of Intuitive Eating within the context of the six paramitas: guiding principles from the Buddhist tradition that support living with clarity, compassion, and purpose. These principles—generosity, discipline, patience, exertion, meditation, and wisdom—serve as essential supports for cultivating a mindful and intuitive relationship with food and your body.

In this workbook, rather than framing the entire process within the paramitas, we will highlight throughout where these elements naturally fit as you move through each chapter of the Intuitive Eating Ecosystem. Every chapter—Soil, Sun, Rain, Trunk, Branches, Air—will illuminate where the paramitas offer guidance and support.

For example, the foundational work of nourishing the soil is deeply rooted in generosity—giving yourself permission to meet your basic needs without guilt. It also involves patience as you build consistent habits, and joyful effort as you engage in self-care, even when it feels challenging.

As you progress through the workbook, notice where these guiding principles show up naturally in your practice. They are not rigid rules or steps—they are companions that support you as you rebuild your relationship with your body.

The Six Paramitas: A Recap

Generosity is the practice of giving freely without expecting anything in return. In the context of Intuitive Eating, it means allowing yourself to have enough—enough food, pleasure, rest, and care—because you are inherently worthy of receiving.

Discipline is the commitment to making choices that align with your values and well-being, not out of punishment, perfectionism, or rigidity but out of self-respect. In Intuitive Eating, this involves discerning what you are feeling and what you need in any given moment so your actions can align with the truth. Discipline also involves coming back to the present moment again and again to reorient yourself.

Patience is the willingness to be with discomfort without rushing to fix or control it. In the Intuitive Eating journey, it means allowing time for healing, honoring setbacks as part of growth, and showing yourself compassion when things feel messy or slow.

Exertion (joyful effort) is the willingness to engage wholeheartedly with what supports your well-being, even when it feels challenging. In Intuitive Eating, it means showing up for yourself consistently—not from obligation but from a desire to care for your body and spirit.

Meditation is the practice of cultivating awareness and being present with your experience as it is. In Intuitive Eating, it means being mindful of your hunger, fullness, and emotions, allowing you to respond rather than react to your body's signals.

Wisdom is the ability to see things clearly, beyond fear or ingrained beliefs, and to act from that deeper knowing. In Intuitive Eating, it means developing panoramic awareness of yourself and your environment so that you can notice trends inside and around you, question diet culture narratives, trust your body's innate guidance, and embrace your own evolving truth.

These paramitas are not isolated practices but interconnected supports. They will appear throughout the workbook to remind you how to approach and sustain this life-long journey. As you build your strong, authentic voice and learn to trust your body, allow these principles to be your steady companions.

Common Concerns and Fears

If you're feeling uncertain about Intuitive Eating, you're not alone. Some common fears include:

- What if I can't hear my hunger or fullness cues?
- What if I still want to lose weight?
- What if I have food rules that feel impossible to break?

These fears are normal. You don't need to have all the answers right now. This workbook will help you gently explore these concerns with curiosity rather than judgment.

A Practice Rooted in Compassion

This journey asks you to abandon black-and-white thinking and embrace the complexity of life. It means learning to dance with discomfort, uncertainty, and change. It's about deepening your self-awareness, your capacity for expression, and your ability to listen and communicate with compassion—not just toward others, but toward yourself.

Like any practice, Intuitive Eating requires patience. And when patience feels hard, self-compassion will be your anchor. It's okay to stumble. In fact, that's how you grow. Your Intuitive Eating path—like your life—is unfolding in each moment, shaped by every thought, choice, breath, and bite.

Hold These Truths Close

As you move through this workbook, I invite you to hold these truths close:

- **Real change happens over time**—not through perfection, but through small, consistent choices to move in a new direction.
- **Your thoughts are habits**—when you catch yourself being unkind, use that moment as an opportunity to practice self-compassion.
- **Celebrate small victories**—even noticing a thought is a triumph. These moments add up.
- **You are always changing**—even when progress feels slow, trust that growth is happening beneath the surface.
- **Obstacles are not failures**—they are lessons in disguise.
- **Reflection is powerful**—take time to honor your progress and the work you're doing.

You Are Not Alone

This work is your gift to yourself. It's an act of self-care, a reclamation of your autonomy, and a path back to trust. And you are not alone in this. Let's walk this journey together.

The Soil: Foundational Needs

This is where your journey begins. Without enough sleep, food, safety, and nervous system regulation, nothing else can take root. The soil represents your most basic creaturely needs—the conditions that allow you to germinate and grow into a deeper understanding of yourself.

The Soil: Foundational Needs

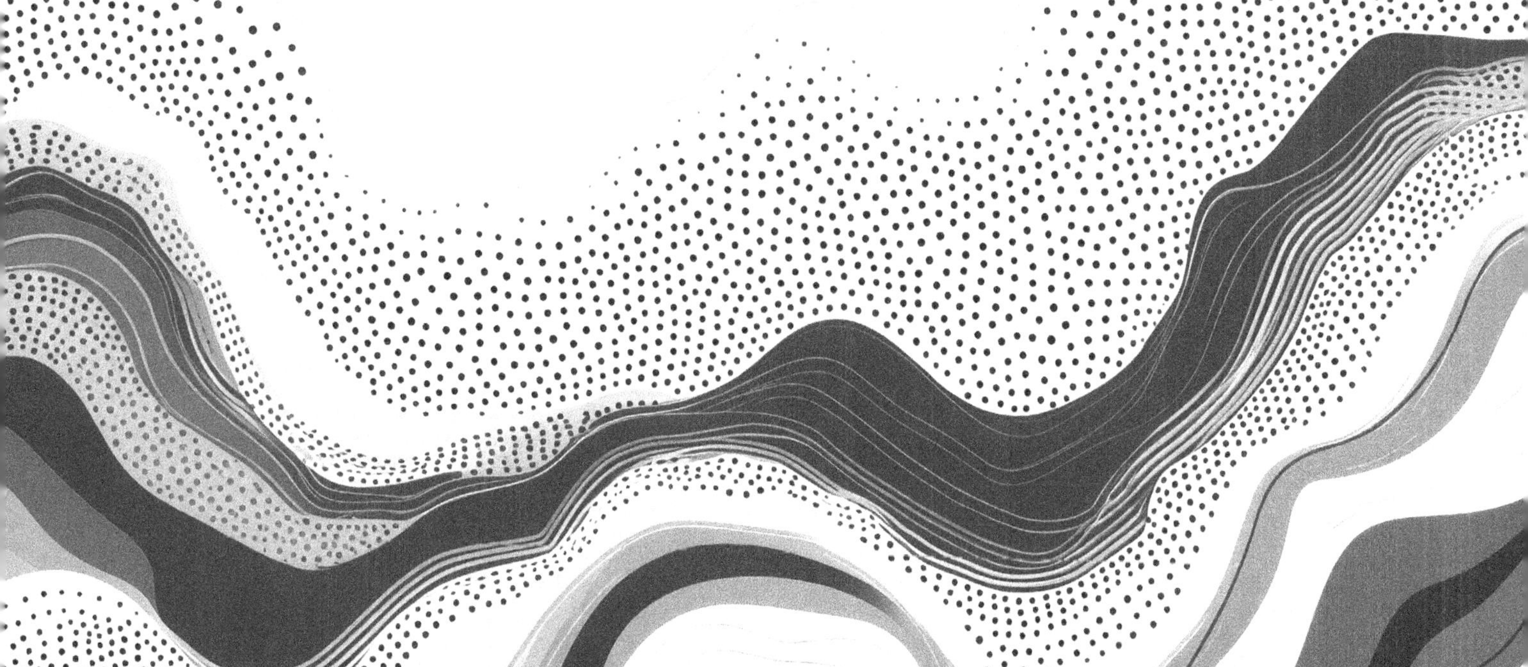

The Paramitas (the how)

> **Generosity:** *I allow myself enough—nourishment, rest, connection, and gentleness.*

> **Discipline:** *I return to what's true, aligning action with respect.*

Patience: I honor slow growth and meet setbacks with compassion.

> **Exertion:** *I show up for myself with joyful, steady effort.*

Meditation: I rest with what is, without fixing or fleeing.

Wisdom: I see clearly and act from clarity and compassion.

This chapter lays the groundwork for your Intuitive Eating journey.

Like any living thing, your ability to grow and thrive depends on your environment. Before we can talk about satisfaction or tending to emotions, we must first ensure the conditions for trust and awareness are present.

In this chapter, you'll explore foundational practices—like getting adequate sleep, nourishing yourself consistently, tending to your nervous system, fostering connection, and respecting your body through comfort and care. These are the roots of the Intuitive Eating Ecosystem. Come back to this chapter anytime you feel untethered; the soil always deserves tending.

You'll practice:

- Noticing, assessing, and adjusting to meet your basic needs
- Feeling and deepening your understanding of your unique hunger experience
- Body respect as a form of self-love

What to Remember When You're Struggling

1. **Real, lasting change takes time and repetition.** Neuroplasticity shows us that transformation isn't instant—it's a practice.
2. **Your ability to grow depends on meeting your basic needs.** Rest, nourishment, hydration, stress management, and safety create the foundation for new thoughts, decisions, and actions.
3. **When those needs aren't met, self-compassion is your best ally.** If you stumble, be gentle with yourself. Return when you can—without judgment.

What would you like to remember in the most challenging moments on your Intuitive Eating journey?

Get the Sleep You Need

Sleep is not a luxury—it's essential nourishment. The National Sleep Foundation recommends that adults get seven to nine hours of sleep each night, not as a rigid rule, but as a daily act of self-trust and care. Here are some ways to support deep, restorative sleep with kindness and intention:

1. Plan for the Rest You Deserve

- Create a consistent sleep rhythm. Your body thrives on routine. Getting to bed and waking up about the same time each night and day helps many people regulate their sleep.
- Protect your rest time. Honor your limits, even when Netflix begs you to stay up.
- Make your space inviting. Cool, dark, and quiet often works best.

2. Avoid Habits That Disrupt Sleep

- Be mindful of caffeine in the afternoon.
- Compassionately check in about alcohol—while it may feel relaxing, it can interrupt deep rest.
- Give screens a curfew. Try turning them off at least an hour before bed.

3. Honor Your Changing Sleep Needs

- Sleep changes with seasons, hormones, stress, and life events.
- Adjust with kindness. If you notice sleep changes, meet them with curiosity rather than frustration. Ask, *What would support my sleep today?*

Reflection:

What are you doing right now to prioritize sleep (i.e., to get seven to nine hours per night)?

What one or two things could you improve to support your sleep?

After a few weeks of trying new habits, what do you notice?

What challenges remain?

Additional Support for Better Sleep

Relaxation Techniques

- **Progressive Muscle Relaxation:** Start at your toes and work your way up, tensing and relaxing each muscle group. This helps release physical tension that might be keeping you awake.
- **Guided Imagery (try the free Insight Timer app):** Picture a peaceful place, like a beach or a forest, and imagine yourself there, engaging all five senses to enhance relaxation. The free Insight Timer, which can be downloaded from an app store, contains many guided meditations and other offerings specifically for sleep.
- **Soothing Sounds:** White (pink, brown, green) noise, nature sounds, or calming music can create a restful atmosphere conducive to sleep.

Which technique seems aligned with you?
Try it and reflect on the results:

Breathwork

- **Four-Seven-Eight Breathing:** Inhale for four seconds, hold for seven, and exhale for eight. This technique can calm the nervous system and promote sleep.
- **Box Breathing:** Inhale for four seconds, hold for four, exhale for four, hold for four. This method helps to slow down thoughts and reduce stress.
- **Diaphragmatic Breathing:** Breathe deeply into your belly rather than shallowly into your chest to encourage relaxation.

Which type of breathwork seems aligned with you?
Try it and reflect on the results:

Meditation

- **Body Scan:** Focus on each part of your body, noticing tension and consciously relaxing.
- **Loving-Kindness:** Send positive thoughts to yourself and others, reducing stress that may interfere with sleep.
- *Shamatha–vipashyana:* See Chapter 6 for full instructions on how to practice this open-eye breath-awareness technique.

Which meditation seems aligned with you?
Try it and reflect on the results:

Cognitive Behavioral Therapy for Insomnia (CBT-I)

- **Challenge negative thoughts:** If you find yourself thinking, *I'll never get to sleep*, try replacing it with a more neutral thought, like, *I can rest even if I don't fall asleep right away*.
- **Reserve bed for sleep and sex only:** Only use your bed for sleep (and sex), to strengthen the brain's association between bed and rest.
- **Try sleep restriction if needed:** Limiting the time spent in bed to the actual amount of sleep you're getting (and not taking afternoon naps that might interfere with nighttime sleep) can improve sleep efficiency.
- Work with a CBT-I provider (see https://cbti.directory/).

Which CBT-I technique seems aligned with you?
Try it and reflect on the results:

Melatonin

- **When it may help:** Melatonin is useful for adjusting sleep cycles, especially when dealing with jet lag, shift work, or delayed sleep phase disorder.
- **Best practices:** A small dose (0.5–3 mg) taken 30–60 minutes before bed (when appropriate) can be effective. More isn't necessarily better.

My approach to mindful melatonin use (optional):

Medications

- **Over-the-counter options:** Antihistamines (e.g., diphenhydramine) may help occasionally but can cause grogginess the next day.
- **Prescription medications:** If sleep struggles persist, a doctor may recommend short-term use of sleep aids like zolpidem (Ambien) or eszopiclone (Lunesta).
- **Considerations:** Medications should be used cautiously, and typically as a last resort, as they can lead to dependency if not managed properly.

My approach to mindful sleep medications (optional):

Before You Move On

If you're not getting enough sleep, it's not a personal failure—it's a signal that something needs care. Rest is not a luxury; it's a biological necessity. Expecting ourselves to function, focus, or grow without adequate sleep is not just unrealistic—it's inhumane. Your healing, your clarity, your ability to nourish and trust yourself all begin with rest. If sleep is a struggle, give it your attention with the same tenderness you would offer a tired child. You deserve that kind of care.

Consistent Nourishment

Your body is not a machine. It can't "fuel up" once and run for hours. You need consistent, compassionate nourishment to regulate energy, mood, and focus. For many, this means eating every few hours and not going longer than four hours without food.

Interoception is your body's ability to sense and interpret internal signals—like hunger, fullness, thirst, fatigue, and emotion. When you eat consistently, you give your body the safety and predictability it needs to communicate those signals more clearly. Structured eating—gently planning meals and snacks throughout the day—can act like scaffolding, helping rebuild your connection to those cues until interoception becomes more reliable and intuitive. Here's an example:

[6:00 am] <u>Wake</u>

[7:00 am] <u>Breakfast</u>

[10:00 am] <u>Snack</u>

[1:00 pm] <u>Lunch</u>

[4:00 pm] <u>Snack</u>

[7:00 pm] <u>Dinner</u>

[10:00 pm] <u>Snack</u>

[10:30 pm] <u>Bed</u>

This is by no means the right pattern for everyone. If you sleep later and breakfast isn't until 9 am, for example, perhaps you don't need that morning snack. If you tend to eat dinner later than 7 pm, perhaps the evening snack isn't necessary. I personally often eat a series of snacks throughout the day instead of larger meals, until I go to visit family in Sicily, and then I adapt to the rhythm there, which is a small breakfast and a larger lunch and dinner.

The point of any structured eating approach is to work with your usual schedule, to not go too long without eating, and to pay attention to the physical sensations that start to emerge. Ultimately, you can remove the "scaffolding" of the structured eating and allow your hunger signals to drive when you eat.

Use this page to create your own personalized plan. If you need multiple structured plans for different days (e.g., weekday vs. weekend day, or workday vs. non-workday), create exactly what you need.

Structured eating plan #1

[　　] ______________

[　　] ______________

[　　] ______________

[　　] ______________

[　　] ______________

[　　] ______________

[　　] ______________

[　　] ______________

Structured eating plan #2

[　　] ______________

[　　] ______________

[　　] ______________

[　　] ______________

[　　] ______________

[　　] ______________

[　　] ______________

[　　] ______________

Structured eating plan #3

[　　] ______________

[　　] ______________

[　　] ______________

[　　] ______________

[　　] ______________

[　　] ______________

[　　] ______________

[　　] ______________

Honor Your Hunger

Hunger exists on a continuum, with not hungry (1 on the scale below) at one end and primally hungry (10 on the scale below) at the other. Many people find food most pleasurable—that is, the brain experiences the greatest "reward" while eating—when gently to moderately hungry (levels 3–5). The ideal hunger level to start eating is when you're hungry enough that food tastes good, but not so hungry that eating feels urgent and mindless.

Use the scale below to start exploring your personal hunger spectrum.

1 Absence of hunger; food might not taste as rewarding as when you're hungry.

2 Slightest hint of hunger emerging.

3 Gentle hunger signals start to emerge: mild hunger pangs, soft rumbling in the stomach.

4 Sensations start to get stronger.

5 Moderate hunger is when food tends to taste best and to feel the most rewarding to the brain. At hunger levels 4–5, you might notice you're more able to sense what you're hungry for, to eat with enjoyment, to notice the sensory qualities of food, and to be aware of emerging fullness. Sensations include gurgling and grumbling in your stomach, aching in your throat or esophagus, thoughts drifting to food and eating.

6 Slightly stronger signals of moderate hunger.

7 Hunger starts to tip over into a more extreme range.

8 Extreme hunger levels such as 7–10 tend to be a stressor to the body. Thoughts might drift to food and eating, concentration is compromised, irritability may arise, you might notice a headache.

9 Not the highest level of hunger, but pretty close.

10 At the level of hunger that is the greatest you've ever felt, you might find it difficult to discern what would satisfy you, and there is a much greater likelihood of eating fast, overeating, and missing out on the pleasures of eating. Eating may also tip over into a binge. Sensations may include pain in the stomach or behind the ribcage, nausea, headache, irritability, dizziness, lightheadedness.

Fill in the scale below to better clarify what hunger feels like in your body:

1 ______________________________________

2 ______________________________________

3 ______________________________________

4 ______________________________________

5 ______________________________________

6 ______________________________________

7 ______________________________________

8 ______________________________________

9 ______________________________________

10 ______________________________________

Reflection:

What do you notice about the progression of hunger in your body?

What do you notice about the connection between hunger level and pleasure while eating?

At what hunger level do you enjoy food the most?

At what level of hunger do you tend to start eating, and how does that affect your eating experience?

Practicing Body Respect

Treating your body with respect, care, and love isn't something you earn—it's something you are inherently worthy of, right now. This is not about self-improvement. It's about meeting yourself as you are and creating conditions in which your body can feel safe, honored, and at home.

Every time you respond to your hunger, drink a glass of water, or choose clothes that feel good on your skin, you are practicing body respect. These small acts are the foundation of healing your relationship with food and yourself.

But respect goes far beyond what we eat. It's how we tend to our needs, how we care for our pain, and how we acknowledge the reality of our lived experience.

Body respect is not a reward for weight loss. It's not conditional. It's a way of saying to yourself, *I matter. This body, today, matters.*

Even unexpected choices—like switching to a softer pair of jeans, pausing a conversation to check in with your breath, or canceling an appointment to get more rest—can be profound acts of body respect.

Tending to Mental Health

Your emotional well-being directly impacts your ability to tune into your body. When anxiety floods your system or depression dulls your senses, interoceptive awareness is compromised—not because you're doing anything wrong, but because your system is working overtime to cope.

Tending to your mental well-being may include:

- Seeking therapy or support for depression, anxiety, trauma, bipolar disorder, or other specific needs
- Exploring medication options when needed
- Allowing yourself rest when emotional overwhelm arises

Honoring Neurodivergence and Sensitivities

If you live with ADHD, OCD, autism spectrum disorder, or synesthesia, or you identify as a highly sensitive person (HSP), your body may process stimuli and needs differently. That doesn't make your experience wrong—it means you may need creative, personalized ways to care for yourself.

Body respect for neurodivergent folks might include:

- Structured routines to support eating and rest
- Minimizing sensory overload (e.g., choosing soft fabrics, noise-reducing tools)
- Creating environments that reduce decision fatigue

Creating Physical Comfort

Your body deserves to feel good in its space. While comfort is often dismissed as indulgent, it's actually a requirement for tuning in. If your waistband is digging into your belly or your mattress is hurting your back, it's no wonder your body's signals get silenced.

Ways to create physical comfort:

- Clothing that fits and feels good
- Furniture that supports your body
- Lighting that soothes rather than stimulates
- Temperature and textures that help you settle

What small changes could make your physical environment
more comfortable?

Prioritizing Preventive Care

Going to the doctor may feel daunting, especially if you've had negative or weight-biased experiences. But advocating for your health is a radical act of body respect. This includes:

- Regular checkups (primary care provider, gynecologist, eye doctor, dentist)
- Screenings (mammograms, colonoscopies, labs)
- Asking questions and advocating for yourself in appointments

What health appointments or screenings do you want to schedule in the next three to six months?

What questions do you have for your healthcare provider(s)?

Body Gratitude: A Daily Practice

You don't have to love your body—or every part of it—to begin a relationship of care. Gratitude is one of the most powerful ways to shift out of self-criticism and into connection.

This isn't about ignoring pain, discomfort, or the very real frustrations you might feel in your body. It's about broadening the lens—acknowledging what your body *does* for you, even in the smallest ways.

You might thank your eyes for helping you notice beauty.

Your hands for holding the ones you love.

Your legs for carrying you through the day.

Your skin for protecting you.

Your breath for anchoring you.

When you practice this kind of gratitude—gently, regularly—you begin to build trust. And trust is one of the deepest forms of body respect.

Try this each day for a week:

Today, I'm grateful for my: _______________________________

Because: ____

Let this practice be simple, honest, and yours. Notice how you feel after a few days of offering thanks—not to perfect your body, but to be in relationship with it.

Body Respect Also Looks Like ...

- Saying no to people, spaces, and expectations that harm you
- Taking your meds without shame
- Allowing joy, pleasure, and rest
- Reaching out for connection when isolation creeps in

Keeping Body Respect Going

This is not a one-time effort. Body respect is a practice you return to again and again, refining as your needs and life evolve. Sometimes, you'll fall out of practice—that's okay. The invitation is always to return. Gently. Honestly. Without shame.

Nervous System Regulation: The Ground Beneath Awareness

You cannot build new habits, connect with hunger cues, or make compassionate choices if your nervous system is stuck in survival mode. Before awareness comes safety. Before change comes regulation.

That's where polyvagal theory comes in. Described by Dr. Stephen Porges—but long present in many indigenous cultures—this theory helps us understand how our nervous systems constantly assess whether we are safe or in danger. This process, called neuroception, happens automatically, below the level of conscious awareness.

When your body perceives safety, it allows for connection, presence, digestion, rest, and trust in bodily signals. But when it detects threats (even subtle or chronic ones), it may shift into:

- Fight or flight (mobilized, anxious, tense, reactive)
- Freeze or shutdown (numb, foggy, disconnected, collapsed)

Neither state is wrong. These are protective responses—brilliant, ancient strategies for survival. But when they persist, they interfere with interoception, your ability to feel hunger, fullness, and emotion clearly.

That's why nervous system regulation is not just supportive of Intuitive Eating—it's essential.

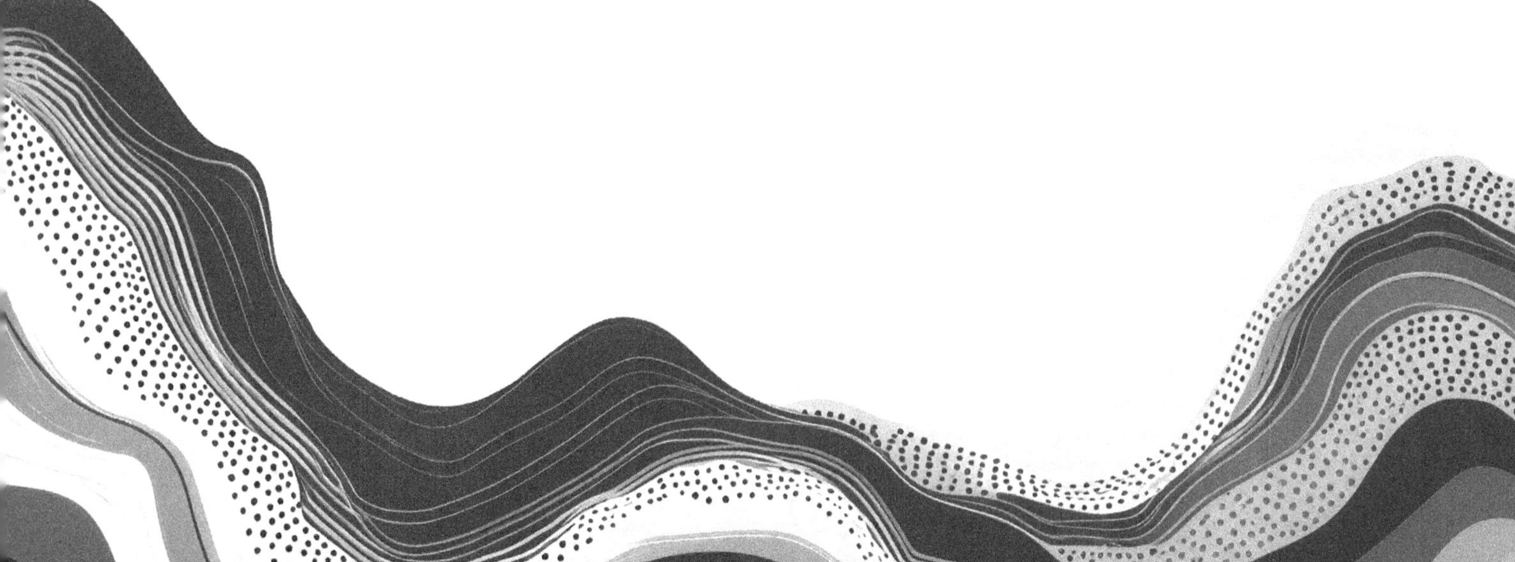

Understanding Your Nervous System States

Your nervous system moves between three main states. The goal is not to stay in one state all the time but to increase your ability to **recognize** and **respond** with compassion.

Ventral Vagal: Safety and Connection

This is your regulated state.

- You feel grounded, present, and connected.
- You're able to listen to your body and respond with care.
- Eating feels calm, mindful, and nourishing.
- You feel curious and open—even when things are uncertain.

Sympathetic: Fight or Flight

This is your mobilized, reactive state.

- You feel anxious, wired, tense, irritable, overwhelmed.
- You may overthink food choices or feel urgency around eating.
- Your body may feel restless or agitated.
- You might reach for food to soothe or distract.

Dorsal Vagal: Freeze or Shutdown

This is your collapsed, disconnected state.

- You feel numb, foggy, tired, or like you're "not here."
- You may not feel hunger or fullness cues at all.
- You might skip meals, feel apathetic, or zone out while eating.
- You feel alone, withdrawn, or hopeless.

Know Your Signs

Everyone's nervous system expresses these states differently. Learning your own cues is a powerful act of self-trust.

Reflection:

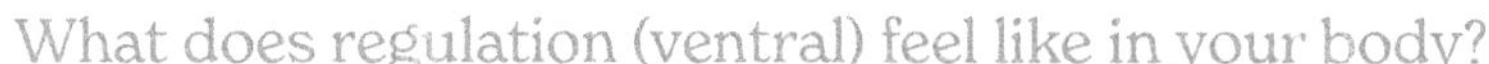

What does regulation (ventral) feel like in your body?

What does fight-or-flight (sympathetic) feel like in your body?

What does shutdown (dorsal) feel like in your body?

Create Your Menu of Supportive Responses

When you notice you're in a sympathetic or dorsal state, it's helpful to have a personalized "menu" of gentle responses to help you shift toward regulation.

Use this space to begin building your own menu.
Try to include at least one option in each of these categories:

Soothing touch (e.g., hand on heart, holding a warm mug):

Breath or body movement (e.g., slow exhale, stretching, walking):

Grounding or sensory tools (e.g., favorite scent, textured object, calming playlist):

Social support or co-regulation (e.g., texting a friend, petting your dog):

Restorative rituals (e.g., making tea, lying on the floor, stepping outside):

Keep this menu somewhere accessible. Add to it as you discover what works for you. No one tool works every time, and that's okay. This is about tending to your nervous system with kindness and curiosity.

We Are Not Meant to Do This Alone: Community, Connection, and Belonging

Healing your relationship with food—and with yourself—can feel deeply personal, but it's not meant to be solitary. We heal best in connection, when we're seen, heard, and supported. Just as disconnection can deepen pain, belonging can be the soil where trust and resilience grow.

You don't need a huge network. One safe relationship—a friend, a partner, a mentor, a support group—can offer profound co-regulation and companionship on this path.

And if you feel like you don't have that right now, know this: the need for connection is not a weakness. It's human. You're allowed to seek it, name it, and nurture it.

Reflection:

Who makes you feel safe, seen, and supported?

When do you feel most like yourself? Who are you with?
What are you doing?

What is one small way you can nurture a sense of connection
this week—through a conversation, a text, a shared meal, or
joining a group?

Where in your life could you invite more belonging—less
performance, more honesty?

What kind of support do you long for?
How might you begin to look for it?

Chapter 1 Key Takeaways

- Foundational needs come first. Before growth can happen, your body and nervous system must feel safe, nourished, and rested.
- Sleep is not a luxury—it's essential. Prioritize both the quantity and the quality of your rest as an act of self-respect.
- Eating consistently rebuilds body trust. Structured eating can gently support your hunger cues until interoception becomes more reliable.
- Interoception is your inner compass. Your ability to sense hunger, fullness, and emotions depends on a regulated, nourished body.
- Your nervous system sets the tone. Regulation—not perfection—is what helps you stay present, responsive, and self-compassionate.
- Learn your patterns of dysregulation. Understanding your nervous system states gives you more choice in how you respond.
- You can build a toolkit that works for you. Breathwork, grounding, co-regulation, and rest are all ways to support safety from the inside out.
- Body respect is a daily practice. Comfort, pleasure, medical care, and mental health support are not rewards—they are your right.
- Gratitude opens the door to trust. Thanking your body—even in small ways—helps shift the focus from criticism to connection.
- We are not meant to do this alone. Connection and belonging are essential. Healing happens more easily when you feel supported.
- This is a cycle, not a checklist. You will return to this foundation again and again. That's not backsliding—it's wisdom.

The Sun: Cognitive Shifts

This is the light that supports your inner transformation. Here, you begin to soften rigid thinking, challenge the food police, and unlearn the diet mentality. The sun shines through nuance and complexity, helping you think differently, with more flexibility, compassion, and truth.

Chapter 2.

The Sun: Cognitive Shifts

The Paramitas (the how)

Generosity: I allow myself enough—nourishment, rest, connection, and gentleness.

> *Discipline: I return to what's true, aligning action with respect.*

> *Patience: I honor slow growth and meet setbacks with compassion.*

Exertion: I show up for myself with joyful, steady effort.

Meditation: I rest with what is, without fixing or fleeing.

> *Wisdom: I see clearly and act from clarity and compassion.*

In the Intuitive Eating Ecosystem, the sun represents the cognitive shifts that illuminate your path forward.

This chapter is about shining a light on the thoughts and beliefs you've inherited and internalized—from diet culture, societal expectations, past experiences, and those actively competing for your attention and dollars. As you become aware of the stories you hold about eating, food, and your body, you gain the ability to discern outside voices from your own inner knowing.

This chapter is not just about finding your voice; it's about clarifying, strengthening, and trusting it. Your authentic voice is rooted in truth, compassion, and lived experience. It knows how to listen, question, discern, and decide—helping you move through a noisy, demanding world with courage and self-trust.

But for many of us, that voice has been dimmed or drowned out. Diet culture, black-and-white thinking, and internalized food rules don't just shape how we eat—they rob us of vital parts of ourselves:

- Our ability to trust our own bodies—to believe that hunger is valid, that fullness can be honored, that pleasure is not a danger.
- Our bodily autonomy—the right to choose what, when, and how we eat, without shame or outside interference.
- Our confidence in our own judgment—replaced by second-guessing, Googling, obsessing, apologizing.
- Our ability to be "certain enough"—to say, *This is right for me right now*, without needing to justify or perfect it.
- Our sense of resilience—the quiet knowing that no matter what happens, we can meet it. We can adjust, recover, and begin again.

Instead, many of us have been left with fear, anxiety, obsession, and the burden of being a "good girl"—always perfect, pleasing, and palatable. We're left with conflicting food rules, mental noise, and self-doubt. In some cases, this cognitive dissonance has even led to disordered eating or mental illness as we try to live up to rules that never truly served us.

This chapter is about reclaiming your light.

Rebuilding your strong, authentic voice doesn't mean you'll never feel doubt again. It means you'll have the tools to move through it with discernment and clarity. You'll learn how to respond to mental noise with compassion, to criticism with care, and to yourself with gentleness.

Because your voice was never really gone—it's just been waiting for the sun to come back.

In this chapter, you will practice:

- Resisting the oversimplification of black-and-white thinking
- Rejecting the diet mentality (especially as it shapeshifts)
- Challenging internal and external "food police"
- Communicating your needs and boundaries nonviolently
- Reclaiming your power through discernment and compassionate skepticism

Setting Your Intention: Reclaiming Your Authentic Voice

Before diving into the work of strengthening your authentic voice, take a moment to set an intention. This is about envisioning the kind of voice you want to develop—not just how it sounds, but how it feels to express yourself with truth, courage, and clarity.

Imagine This

Close your eyes and picture a version of yourself who speaks confidently and kindly—both to yourself and to others. Imagine a voice that is clear, steady, and grounded. One that knows how to say *yes* and *no* without feeling guilty. One that questions harmful messages without being shaken. One that honors your body and your needs without apology.

When you picture this voice, ask yourself:

- What words does it choose?
- How does it sound—gentle, firm, joyful, calm?
- What does it feel like in your body to speak this way?
- How would this voice change how you move through your day?
- How would it influence your relationship with food and your body?

Write Your Intention

In the space below, describe the authentic voice you are committed to cultivating. Don't worry about getting it perfect—just let your words flow.

My intention for my authentic voice is to:

This voice will help me:

A phrase I can return to when I feel uncertain is:

As you move through this chapter, revisit this intention whenever you feel disconnected or overwhelmed. Your voice is not something you have to invent—it's already within you. This process is about clearing away what has silenced it and inviting it to grow stronger.

With the seed of that voice in your head, let's begin the cognitive work of a mindful Intuitive Eating path.

Resisting Black-and-White Thinking

Life is rarely either/or. But diet culture thrives on extremes: "good" vs. "bad," "healthy" vs. "unhealthy," "success" vs. "failure." These kinds of rigid categories feel tidy—but they come at a high cost. They lead to shame, rigidity, and ultimately, self-abandonment.

Why are we starting here? Because one of the greatest barriers to body trust is cognitive distortion—when we force complex realities into simple, binary boxes. It's not your fault. We've been taught to see the world this way, especially around food and bodies. But if we want to reclaim our voice and rebuild trust, we must make space for complexity. For nuance. For both/and.

Take a food like a croissant.

- To someone healing from an eating disorder, eating a croissant might be a huge victory—an act of freedom.
- To someone with celiac disease, it could be dangerous.
- To a child in Paris, it's a normal breakfast.
- To someone steeped in diet culture, it might be labeled "bad" or "fattening."
- To someone else, it might be a spiritual experience—warm, flaky, eaten slowly on a park bench.

So, is the croissant good or bad?

Healthy or unhealthy?

Right or wrong?

It depends.

It always depends.

And that's the point. When we try to flatten life into categories, we miss what's really happening. We miss context. We miss humanity. We miss *ourselves*.

When you catch yourself in black-and-white thinking—about food, your body, your progress, your worth—pause and ask:

- What might I be missing here?
- Is there more to this story?
- What would I see if I zoomed out 10,000 feet?

- Could this be both true and incomplete?
- What else could also be true?

This is where your strong, authentic voice begins—not in having the "right" answer, but in being willing to hold more than one truth at a time.

Consider the following:

Where do you notice "either/or" thinking in your food or body beliefs?

What's a recent situation where both/and thinking could have offered more space and self-compassion?

Try reframing one of your black-and-white thoughts into something more flexible and truthful:

1. Original thought:	2. What makes this thought feel true:
3. A more flexible, truthful reframe:	4. How does this new thought feel in your body?

Learning to move beyond black-and-white thinking opens up space for nuance and flexibility. But even when we begin to let go of rigid categories, diet culture can still sneak back in—disguised in new, seemingly reasonable ways. To truly reclaim your voice, it's important to recognize how diet culture shapeshifts and attempts to reinsert itself into your thoughts, even after you've consciously rejected it.

Recognizing the Shapeshifter: A New Way to Spot Diet Culture

One of the most frustrating things about diet culture is that it doesn't always look like a diet. It's a shapeshifter. And just when you think you've left it behind, it reappears in new forms—more subtle, more seductive, more socially acceptable.

It used to be calorie counting, weigh-ins, and low-fat everything. Now, it's "clean eating," intermittent fasting, detoxes, macros, gut health, biohacking, anti-aging regimens, and body "optimization." It tells you it's about health, but at its core, it's still about control—about shrinking yourself, perfecting yourself, fixing yourself. It just wears different clothes.

Diet culture has gotten smarter. It now co-opts the language of wellness, feminism, empowerment—even Intuitive Eating. It says things like:

- "It's not a diet, it's a lifestyle."
- "I'm just being healthy."
- "Discipline is self-love."
- "I just feel better when I cut out gluten/dairy/sugar/carbs/joy."

The problem is, some of those things might be true for you. And that's what makes this so hard. The question is not, *What does this claim say?* but rather, *How does this claim affect me? What does it do to my thoughts, my body, my nervous system, my sense of self?*

Recognizing diet mentality as it shapeshifts is not about judging your choices. It's about giving you a way to pause and check in—to come back to your own inner compass, especially when the world is shouting conflicting advice.

A Three-Step Check-In to Spot Diet Culture

The next time you encounter a message about food, health, or your body—whether from a doctor, a podcast, a friend, or your own inner voice—try this:

1. Does it align with my values and intuition?
   Does this message resonate with what I believe about bodies, dignity, and care? Or does it contradict what I know, deep down, to be true?
2. How does it make me feel—physically, emotionally, mentally?
   Do I feel anxious, ashamed, obsessed, or unworthy when I hear it? Or do I feel grounded, curious, empowered?
3. If I follow it, what is the real impact on my well-being, both in the short term and in the longer term? How does it affect my energy, my relationships, my freedom, my mental health?

Reflection:

Where have you noticed diet culture wearing a new disguise?
(e.g., clean eating, biohacking)

Where did it show up?
(e.g., social media, wellness podcast, family advice)

Three-Step Check-In:

1. Does it align with my values and intuition?

2. How does it make me feel—physically, emotionally, mentally?

3. What is the honest impact if I follow it?

Write two to three phrases that reinforce your inner skeptic.
(e.g., *That sounds like restriction in a new outfit.* or,
Who profits from me doubting myself?)

Challenging the Food Police: Dismantling the Voices That Distort

If you've ever felt guilty about what you were eating—or what you were considering eating—you've likely encountered the food police. These are the voices, both internal and external, that rush in to judge your choices.

Sometimes, they sound like your own thoughts. Sometimes, they're the echoes of a parent, a doctor, a personal trainer, a wellness influencer, or a partner. These voices can become so loud and constant that they drown out the one voice that matters: your own.

But not all food police are the same. Let's break them down:

External Food Police

These are the people and systems outside of you that monitor, comment on, or try to control what and how you eat.

- "You don't need that."
- "Are you sure you should be eating that?"
- "I'm just worried about your health."

Supposed intention: Concern, care, helpfulness, moral guidance.
Actual effect: Shame, confusion, and erosion of trust in your own judgment.

We'll come back to the External Food Police at the end of this chapter by learning to use nonviolent communication to advocate for yourself. For now, though, let's work with those insidious internal food police that can be so judgmental and disorienting.

Internal Food Police

There's a voice inside you that sounds stern, judgmental, and always ready to remind you when you're not doing things "right." You might think of it as your "responsible self" or your "health-conscious voice"—the part of you that tries to keep you on track. But in reality, this voice often functions as the Internal Food Police—a force that not only monitors your eating but also distorts your relationship with food and your body.

The Internal Food Police often sound like your own thoughts, but they rarely originate from you. These voices are inherited—from family members, diet culture, healthcare professionals, media messages, and even past versions of yourself who were just trying to survive. They've become so deeply embedded that you may not even realize they're not you.

The Harmful Intentions of the Internal Food Police

The Internal Food Police might seem like they're protecting you—from weight gain, from judgment, from perceived failure. They claim to offer control, self-discipline, and improvement. But what they actually do is undermine your autonomy and sense of self-trust.

Common Internal Food Police Messages:

- *You've already had enough.*
- *You're being bad.*
- *You'll regret this later.*
- *You're out of control.*
- *You can't trust yourself around that food.*

Supposed intention: Control, protection, self-discipline, improvement.

Actual effect: Fear, hypervigilance, self-doubt, and disconnection from your body's cues.

The Internal Food Police create a hostile environment where food becomes loaded with moral judgment, performance pressure, and anxiety. You may not know whether you actually like a food, whether you're hungry for it, whether you enjoy it, or whether you feel satisfied after eating. Instead of eating intuitively, you might eat from a place of obedience, fear, or compulsion.

This chapter is about disempowering those voices—not with more rules, but by turning the volume up on your own intuition. It's about getting curious, relearning your preferences, and reclaiming pleasure. You don't have to be at war with food—or with yourself. You can build a relationship with food that is grounded, joyful, and yours.

A Slow Process:
Reducing the Charge

These internal voices didn't form overnight, and they won't disappear quickly either. It takes time to reduce the charge of the most persistent thoughts. You may notice them cropping up even as you do this work—and that's okay. The goal isn't to eliminate them, but to soften them, to recognize them for what they are, and to choose differently.

Think of this as a practice in compassion, not perfection. Each time you notice the Food Police and respond with curiosity rather than judgment, you reclaim a bit more of your autonomy.

Identify Your Internal Food Police

Use the chart below to map out some of your most common critical thoughts. Include both what the voice says and what it really means to you.

Thought	What It Sounds Like	Deeper Fear	Actual Effect on You
You've already had enough.	I'll lose control if I eat more.	Fear of overeating, judgment from others	Anxiety, guilt, eating faster to finish
You're being bad.	I'm failing at being healthy.	Fear of being unworthy or out of control	Shame, desire to restrict later
You'll regret this later.	You're making a mistake you'll pay for.	Fear of consequences, weight gain	Fixation, food guilt, self-criticism
You can't trust yourself.	You're inherently flawed around food.	Fear of never changing	Self-doubt, hypervigilance around eating

Compassionate Responses

Choose one of the thoughts from your list, and practice responding to it in a way that honors your body and rebuilds trust.

Reflection:

Thought:

What is the deeper fear underneath it?

What is your lived experience that challenges this fear?

Compassionate response you'll offer instead:

"I hear you, but I choose to ___________."

Taking a Step Back

Sometimes, the charge of a critical thought can feel overwhelming.
When that happens, take a moment to step back and question its origins.

Reflections:

- Where do you think this voice originally came from?
- What is it trying to protect you from?
- Is this voice helping you live in alignment with your values?
- If it's not, what might you say to reassure this part of you?
- How could you invite more compassion into this conversation?

Ongoing Practice: Reducing the Charge

Every time you encounter the Internal Food Police, treat it as an opportunity to practice discernment. You may not change the thought immediately, but each time you acknowledge it without reacting—without guilt, without shame—you take a small step toward dismantling its power.

When the thought arises again, ask yourself:
- *Is this thought helping or hurting me?*
- *What does my authentic voice say in response?*
- *How can I choose to nourish myself right now—without fear or judgment?*

With practice (it's all about practice), you'll notice that some of the fiercest critical voices start to soften. They may still show up, but their grip on you will loosen. You'll begin to see them not as truths, but as old echoes of stories you no longer need to follow.

Reflection:

External Food Police: Advocating for Yourself with Nonviolent Communication

You deserve to feel safe and empowered in conversations about food, body, and boundaries. Using principles of nonviolent communication (NVC)—observation, feeling, need, and request—you can speak from clarity instead of defensiveness.

Complete the following scripts to practice your voice:

At family dinner:

"When you comment on my plate, I feel _______________________ because I need

_______________________. Would you be willing to _______________________?"

At the doctor's office:

"I'm here for _______________. I've had harmful experiences with weight stigma

in the past, and I'd prefer we focus on _______________ instead of my weight."

When someone comments on your body:

"I know you mean well, but I don't find body talk helpful. Let's talk about something that matters to both of us."

Reflection:

What situations make it hardest for you to speak up? Why?

What values are you protecting when you set a boundary?

What words help you stay rooted when you're feeling vulnerable?

Situation:

Observation (without judgment):

Feeling:

Need:

Request:

What value are you protecting by speaking up?

What support do you need to follow through?

Chapter 2 Key Takeaways

- Intuitive Eating is a lifelong practice. It gets easier with repetition and compassion.
- Diet culture evolves, but so can your ability to spot and reject it.
- Thought work is not about controlling your mind—it's about creating space for truth.
- You don't need to fight the food police. You can simply stop listening.
- Speaking up for yourself is hard—but every time you do, you strengthen the voice that will carry you forward.
- Black-and-white thinking oversimplifies complex experiences and leads to shame, rigidity, and disconnection.
- Embracing "both/and" thinking opens up space for nuance, curiosity, and growth.
- Diet culture often masquerades as wellness, discipline, or optimization—your body's wisdom is a more trustworthy guide.
- The Internal Food Police may sound like you, but their messages often originate from fear-based conditioning.
- Getting curious about your preferences helps you reclaim pleasure and reconnect with your body's cues.
- Disempowering critical thoughts takes time—gentle repetition, lived experience, and compassion are key.
- Using a simple check-in—*Does this align with my values? How does it feel? What is the impact?*—can help you navigate confusing food messaging.
- Nonviolent communication allows you to advocate for yourself with clarity and care, especially in challenging situations.
- Your authentic voice is rooted in lived experience, truth, and self-trust—it may have been quieted, but it has never disappeared.

The Rain: Emotional Nourishment

This is the water that soaks into the roots of your heart. It's the ongoing work of tending to your inner voice—learning to speak to yourself with warmth, honoring your vulnerability, and creating space for your feelings without judgment. This is the realm of self-compassion and emotional bravery.

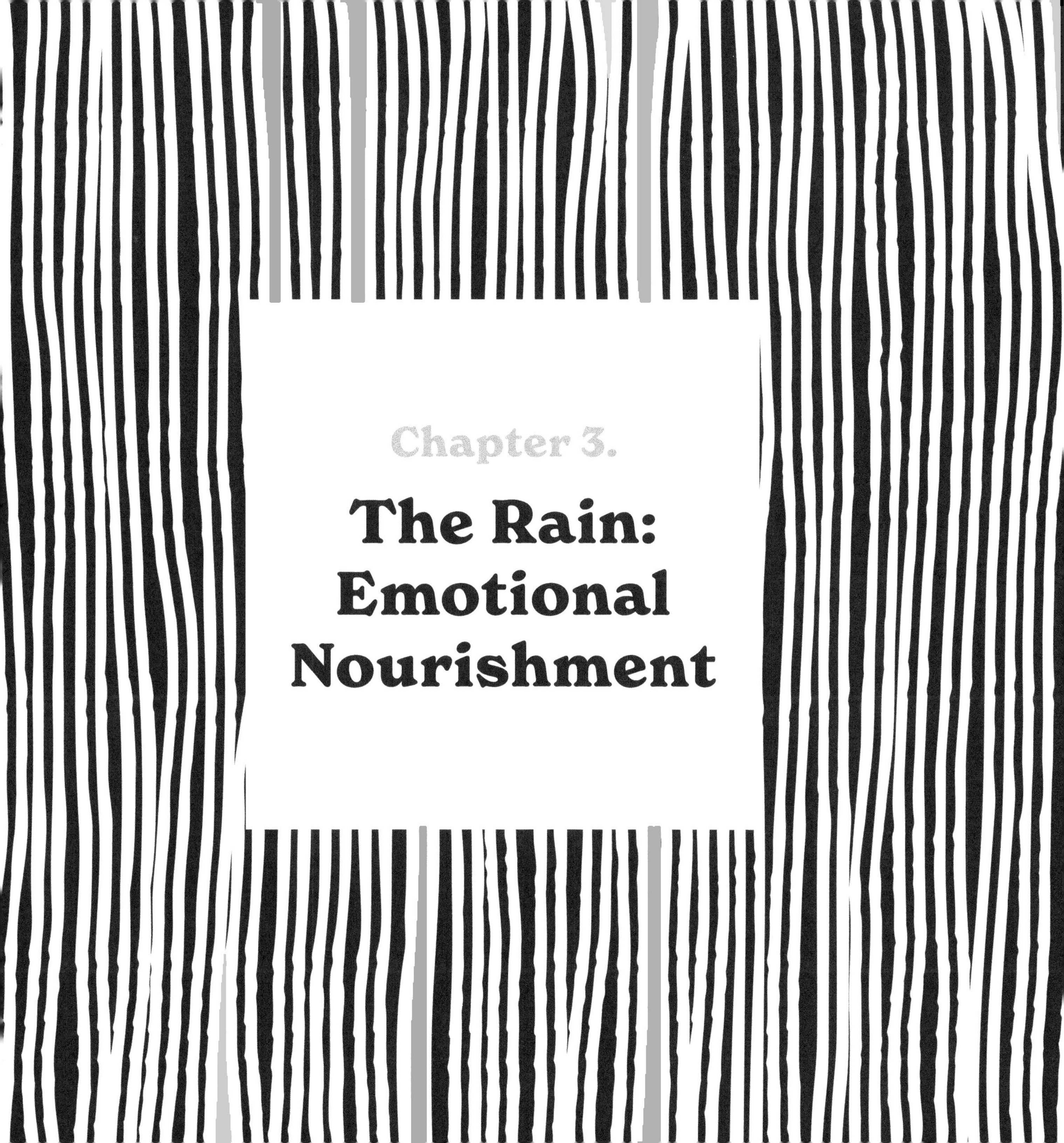

The Rain: Emotional Nourishment

The Paramitas (the how)

> **Generosity:** *I allow myself enough—nourishment, rest, connection, and gentleness.*

Discipline: I return to what's true, aligning action with respect.

> **Patience:** *I honor slow growth and meet setbacks with compassion.*

Exertion: I show up for myself with joyful, steady effort.

> **Meditation:** *I rest with what is, without fixing or fleeing.*

Wisdom: I see clearly and act from clarity and compassion.

Why Emotional Work Matters

This chapter isn't just about emotional eating. It's about coming home to your emotional life.

Once you've begun to meet your basic biological needs—adequate nourishment, rest, safety, and comfort—you're in a better position to face a deeper truth: you are an emotional being. We all are. And just as ignoring physical hunger creates chaos, so does ignoring emotional hunger.

Our culture encourages us to avoid discomfort at all costs. We're taught to bypass pain, spin it into productivity, or reframe it into something more palatable. But avoidance doesn't erase emotion—it only intensifies our suffering, often redirecting it into food, body image, or shame.

We are hard-wired to prefer pleasure over pain. That's not weakness—it's human. But compulsive avoidance of discomfort limits our capacity to fully live. When we allow ourselves to feel the full spectrum of our emotions—not just the "positive" ones—we build resilience, self-trust, and authenticity. Ironically, the more space we make for discomfort, the more vibrant our joy becomes. It's richer. More embodied. More real.

We all eat emotionally. That's not a flaw—it's part of being alive. But when food becomes the *only* way we cope, we lose access to a broader, more empowering toolkit for tending to our hearts.

This chapter is about reclaiming that toolkit. You'll learn how to:

- Recognize and name your emotions
- Understand your nervous system's role in emotional awareness
- Discern what you truly need in moments of distress
- Work with impermanence and emotional arcs
- Embrace emotional eating without shame—and expand your options
- Practice self-compassion as a way of being

Because when you tend to your heart, food becomes one of many forms of care—not a battlefield, not a secret, and not a punishment.

Basic Emotions: Building Your Vocabulary

To tend to your heart, you must first know how to *name* what's there.

Many of us grew up without emotional fluency. We weren't taught how to distinguish sadness from shame, or fear from anger. We may have been praised for suppressing "negative" emotions or punished for expressing them. Our emotional vocabulary shrank—or was never fully developed to begin with.

But emotional awareness is not just about labeling feelings. It's about reclaiming access to the full, nuanced range of human experience. You can't meet your needs if you don't know what you're feeling. And you can't respond to yourself with compassion if all feelings are reduced to "good" or "bad." You're much more wonderfully complex than that!

A helpful tool is the Feelings Wheel (www.feelingswheel.com), which expands basic emotional categories into more specific and complex shades of feeling. You'll find words you already know—and some you've maybe never consciously experienced. That's the point: there are emotions we welcome easily, and others we've never really met. Part of this work is expanding your emotional vocabulary so you can recognize yourself more fully.

Start with these core emotions:

- Anger
- Sadness
- Fear
- Joy
- Disgust
- Surprise
- Shame
- Love

These are the emotional "roots" from which more nuanced feelings grow.

Reflection:

Which of these core emotions do you recognize most easily in yourself?

Which ones feel threatening, shameful, or off-limits?

Are there emotions you tend to avoid, suppress, or numb? Why?

Which emotions have you never really given yourself permission to feel?

Try This:

Visit feelingswheel.com, choose one core emotion (like anger or sadness), and explore the related words.

- What feels familiar?
- What feels foreign?
- What might happen if you made space for *all* of it?

Remember: You don't have to fix or analyze your feelings—just notice them. Naming is an act of awareness. Awareness is the first step toward healing.

Reminder: Foundations First

Before you dive into emotional work, pause and check in with your basic biological needs.

Your ability to feel and work with emotions depends, in part, on how resourced your body is. If you're exhausted, underfed, disconnected, or in physical pain, your system will prioritize survival over introspection. This isn't a flaw—it's your body doing what it was built to do: protect you.

So when emotions feel inaccessible, overwhelming, or strangely absent, ask yourself whether your basic needs have been met. If not, that's the place to start. Give your body the nourishment, rest, and care it needs to create the conditions for emotional awareness to emerge.

If those needs *have* been met and you still feel blocked, that's okay too. It simply reveals where your current edge lies. With gentleness and repeated practice, you may notice new levels of emotional clarity unfolding—just as a flower opens when the conditions are right.

It's also important to acknowledge that unprocessed trauma can make emotional work especially complex. Trauma can fragment awareness, numb sensations, or flood the system with more than it can manage. That's why discernment is crucial: sometimes, it's wise to lean into discomfort, and other times, the most compassionate thing you can do is wait, resource yourself, and return later.

Check-In Prompt:

- Have I eaten enough today?
- Have I had rest and connection?
- Am I safe enough to feel?
- If not, what's one small thing I can do to meet a basic need right now?

You are not behind. You are not failing. You are tending to the ground in which everything else grows.

From Neuroception to Interoception: Laying the Groundwork

Your emotional awareness doesn't start in your mind—it begins in your nervous system.

As we explored in Chapter 1, polyvagal theory teaches us that the body constantly scans the environment for cues of safety or threat. This process—called neuroception—happens automatically, without conscious thought. It's what determines whether you feel calm and connected, anxious and activated, or shut down and disengaged.

When your body senses safety, it shifts into a more regulated state. From this place, mindfulness becomes available. You're no longer just reacting—you're able to pause and notice. And with that mindful awareness, you can begin to access interoception: your capacity to perceive what's happening inside your body in real time.

This might include recognizing hunger or fullness, tightness in your chest, butterflies in your stomach, or a lump in your throat. These physical signals are the early language of emotion. Learning to detect and decipher them is how emotional literacy begins.

Try This Practice:

1. Place one or both hands on your heart or belly.
2. Take three slow, extended exhales—making your out-breath longer than your in-breath.
3. Gently ask yourself:
   What am I feeling in my body right now?
4. Stay curious. No need to name or fix anything yet. Just notice.

Record any reflections here:

This simple practice strengthens your ability to move from unconscious perception (neuroception) to conscious awareness (interoception). It helps you notice when your nervous system is signaling danger—and when it might be safe enough to feel, reflect, and respond.

This is the inner groundwork for working with emotion: not pushing through, but listening closely.

Discernment: What's Really Happening Here?

Strong emotions can blur our vision. They can feel urgent, overwhelming, or impossible to sit with—especially if you've learned to cope by pushing them away, overriding them, or trying to fix them fast.

But discernment asks something different. It's the skill of gently pausing, turning toward your experience, and asking: *What's really going on here?*

In Buddhist practice, discipline (śīla) isn't about punishment or control. It's about returning—again and again—to the present moment and choosing the next wise step. Sometimes, that step is action. Other times, it's just making space for what's here, without running away. In this way, discipline becomes a form of self-respect and responsiveness—a way of being with yourself that is rooted in compassion and care, not force.

From a trauma-informed perspective, discernment also means knowing your edges. If something feels like too much, too soon, that's not a failure—it's information. Your nervous system may be protecting you from overwhelm. In those moments, the "right step" might be soothing your body, grounding, or waiting until you're more resourced.

When you do have capacity, discernment can help you untangle what's at the core of a strong emotion or impulse. Often, what we think is the issue isn't the whole picture.

You might feel anxious, but the deeper emotion is grief.

You might feel rage, but underneath is a boundary that's been crossed.

You might reach for food, but what you really crave is rest, touch, or time alone.

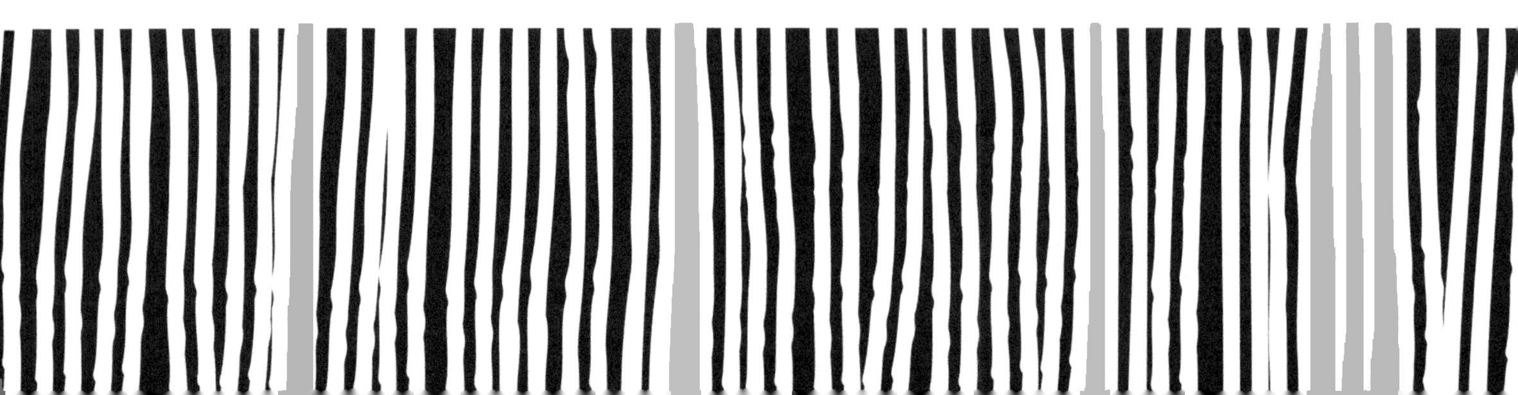

Emotional Decoding Exercise

Try this when you're feeling emotionally stirred up or uncertain about your needs.

What just happened? (Describe the situation briefly):

What emotion do I think I'm feeling?

Can I allow this emotion to be here—just for now?

☐ Yes   ☐ Not yet   ☐ Maybe, with support

If I stay with it a little longer, does another emotion emerge?

What might I really need right now?

☐ Rest   ☐ Creative expression
☐ Connection   ☐ Boundaries
☐ Movement   ☐ Nourishment
☐ Reassurance   ☐ Other: _______

List three kind, feasible ways to meet this need:

1.

2.

3.

Remember: You don't have to get it "right." This isn't about solving your emotions—it's about staying curious. With time and safety, discernment becomes a deeply trustworthy compass.

Impermanence:
The Heart's Hardest Truth

Everything changes. Every breath. Every meal. Every feeling. Every moment. This isn't just poetic—it's biological, neurological, cosmic. It's the truth of being alive.

And depending on your perspective, that might feel like good news, bad news, or something more nuanced.

Impermanence means pain doesn't last forever—but neither does joy. It means you are not stuck, but it also means you can't hold on.

We tend to resist this truth.

We cling to joy, hoping it will stay.

We reject pain, trying to push it away.

But resisting impermanence doesn't stop change—it just adds suffering.

Emotional freedom begins when we stop trying to control the timeline and start riding the natural arc of experience.

Understanding Arcs:
The Anatomy of Experience

Everything we feel, think, or do follows a predictable shape—an arc.

It arises, it peaks, and it dissolves.

This is true whether we're talking about a craving, a conversation, a panic attack, a celebration, or a piece of chocolate cake.

And your *response* to the arc often depends on whether the experience is something you like, dislike, or feel neutral about.

- When we like something, we try to extend the peak and avoid the decline.
- When we dislike something, we try to skip straight to the end.
- And when we're neutral, we may not notice the arc at all.

But here's the paradox: staying with the arc—instead of trying to speed it up or hold it back—is what builds resilience. You learn that you *can* feel something all the way through and come out the other side.

Arcs Exist on Multiple Levels

You'll find them in the micro and the macro.

Micro arcs might include:
- A single breath
- A moment of hunger
- The experience of eating a meal
- A flash of irritation or joy

Macro arcs might include:
- A day or week
- A period of grief or healing
- A job or career
- A chapter of life (early motherhood, perimenopause, recovery, etc.)

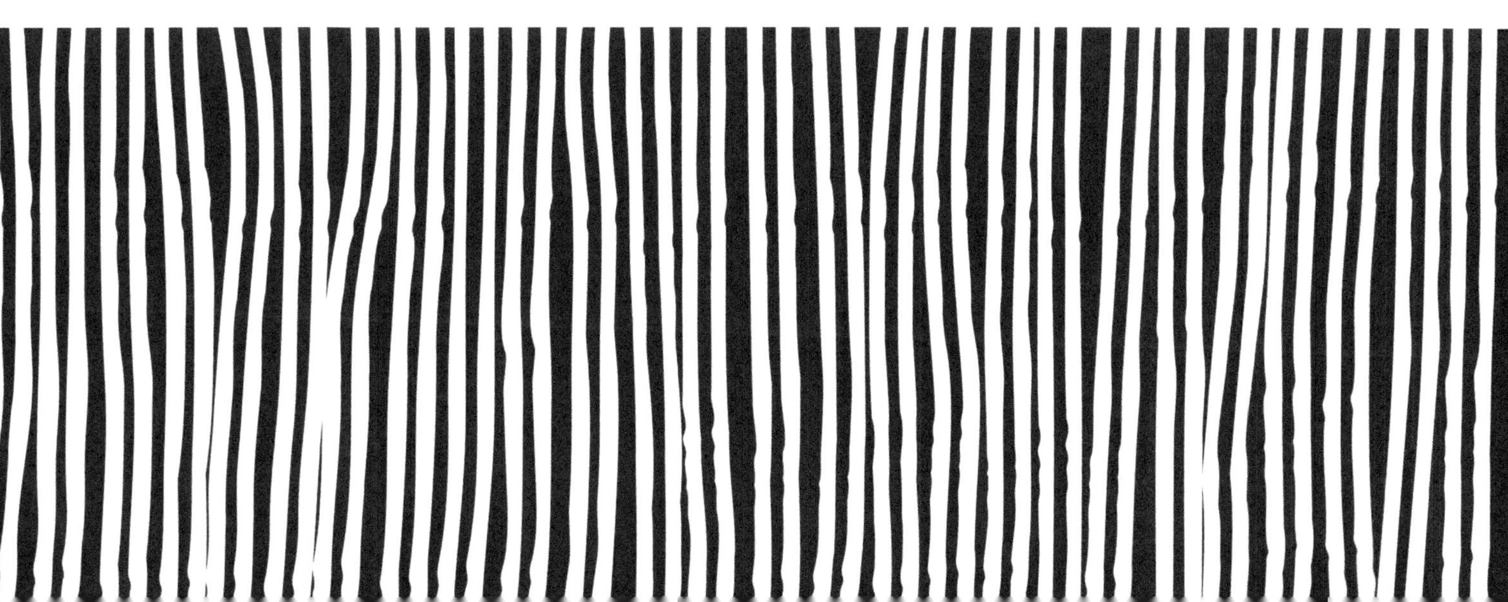

Exercise: Track an Arc

Choose one micro and one macro arc from your life. Observe or reflect on the rise, the peak, and the dissolution of each.

Micro arc example (a craving, an emotion, a moment):

- What triggered its arising?
- What did the peak feel like?
- How did it eventually shift or dissolve?
- What happened when you didn't interrupt the arc?

Macro arc example (a larger transition or experience):

- When did it begin?
- What have been its most intense moments?
- Is it still unfolding, or has it resolved?
- What has it taught you?

Zooming In and Zooming Out

Being with impermanence also means developing dual awareness:

- Zooming in helps you fully feel what's happening.
- Zooming out helps you keep perspective.

Try This Three-Part Reflection:

1. **Zoom In:** What am I feeling in this moment—emotionally, physically, energetically?
2. **Zoom Out:** In the grander arc of this day, week, or season . . . what else is true?
3. **Hold Both:** What shifts when I let both realities be valid?

   How can I honor my experience *and* remember that it will change?

Reminder:

Impermanence isn't something to fear—it's something to *trust*.

Nothing lasts forever, not even this moment.

Which means . . . *you are always in motion*. And that is how we heal.

Emotional Eating: Not the Enemy

Emotional eating has long been villainized—framed as a lack of willpower, a personal failing, or something to be "fixed." But here's the truth: Eating in response to emotions is deeply human. From the moment we're born, we're comforted through food. It's not a glitch in our system—it's part of our wiring.

In fact, the Intuitive Eating approach has evolved alongside this understanding. In earlier editions, the guidance was to "cope with your emotions without using food." But the most recent edition shifts that language meaningfully: "cope with your emotions with kindness." That small change says a lot. It acknowledges that food is *one* way we cope—not the only way, not a wrong way, just one tool among many.

Moralizing emotional eating—thinking of it as "giving in," "being weak," or "failing"—only adds layers of shame and disconnection. Ironically, it's often this shame that drives us further from understanding what we're really feeling or needing in the first place.

Instead, emotional eating can be a clue—a compassionate flag that says, *Something needs tending to here*

What matters is not whether you eat emotionally, but whether you can stay connected to yourself as you do. Whether you can approach the moment with curiosity instead of condemnation. Whether you can develop more options for responding to your emotional needs—not to replace food out of guilt, but to expand your toolkit.

Because there will be times when the warm, familiar comfort of food is exactly right. And there will be other times when what you need is a walk, a deep breath, a nap, a good cry, or a call with a friend. You're allowed to choose.

Reflection: Emotional Eating Inventory

What do I tend to crave when I feel . . .

Sad:

Anxious:

Lonely:

Overwhelmed:

In those moments, what does food offer me?
(Comfort? Numbing? Grounding? Familiarity?)

Does it help? Does it hurt? Does it depend?

Building Your Soothing Menu

Use this space to brainstorm other ways of caring for yourself when emotions run high. (These are *options,* not obligations. There is no moral hierarchy.)

Physical comfort:
(e.g., soft blanket, comfy clothes, stretching, warm bath)

Emotional connection:
(e.g., texting a friend, journaling, hugging a pet)

Sensory support:
(e.g., music, nature sounds, aromatherapy)

Next time you notice the impulse to eat in response to an emotion, ask yourself gently:

Is food what I truly need right now?

If yes, eat with awareness and kindness.

If no—or if you're not sure—pause and get curious.

What else might help right now?

There's no wrong answer. There's just exploration.

Other Hungers: Beyond the Plate

Appetite is not a problem. Desire is not a flaw.

We are creatures of longing—from the moment we're born, we reach for warmth, touch, safety, beauty, and love. These are not indulgences; they are essential parts of being alive. Yet many of us were taught, implicitly or explicitly, that our appetites—especially those not tied to food—were shameful, excessive, or dangerous.

When our desires go unmet, they don't disappear—they get submerged, distorted, and rerouted. Often, they show up in our relationship with food.

And that makes sense.

Food is accessible. It's socially acceptable. It's often tied to reward, comfort, and self-soothing. And unlike other forms of nourishment—intimacy, rest, creativity, belonging—we *must* eat anyway. So, when deeper hungers go unacknowledged or unmet, food may become the only reliable source of satisfaction in our day.

That doesn't make you broken. It makes you *human*.

But when food becomes the primary outlet for all needs—when it bears the full weight of what is unspoken or unfulfilled—our relationship with eating can become tangled in confusion, shame, or guilt.

This part of the journey is about getting curious about your *other* hungers. Learning to name them. Making space for them. And slowly, compassionately, building a more diverse menu of nourishment.

Explore Your Other Hungers

Journaling Prompts:

I feel most alive when . . .

I long for more . . .

I wish someone would really see . . .

When I think of desire, I feel . . .

If I gave myself permission to want, I might discover . . .

Create a Personal Menu of Nourishment

Use this space to reflect on what truly feeds you—not just on the plate, but in your heart, mind, and body. Add real examples to make this list personal and actionable.

Nourishment Category	What You Crave	Examples or Ideas
Connection	To feel understood, supported, seen	A heart-to-heart conversation, a hug, time with a trusted friend
Creativity	To express, explore, build something meaningful	Journaling, singing, crafting, designing, painting, problem-solving
Movement	To inhabit and enjoy your body	Dancing, walking outdoors, stretching, swimming, yoga
Spirituality	To feel connected to something greater	Meditation, prayer, time in nature, ritual, awe-inspiring art or music
Pleasure	To feel delight, sensuality, or joy	A warm bath, delicious scent, candlelight dinner, soft clothes, great sex
Rest	To slow down, reset, and recover	Naps, unstructured time, saying no, sleep, solitude
Play	To feel free, curious, and light	Games, improv, laughter, pets, spontaneous adventures
Purpose	To feel useful, needed, or clear in your values	Volunteering, meaningful work, creating something for others
Beauty	To be surrounded by what feels life-affirming	Flowers, poetry, design, color, music, sunlight, water, fresh air

Reflection:

Which of these hungers have been going unmet?

How might tending to one of them soften the pressure you've placed on food?

Self-Compassion: The Ultimate Practice

Self-compassion isn't a luxury—it's a lifeline. When you're navigating emotional eating, intense feelings, unmet needs, or frustration with your current reality, compassion isn't just helpful. It's essential.

Without self-compassion, we tend to double down on shame, spiraling into old beliefs like *I'm too much*, *I should be past this*, or *What's wrong with me?* These thoughts don't help. They isolate. They paralyze. And they pull you away from your own wisdom.

But compassion changes the air around you. It creates the conditions where truth can emerge—not in judgment, but in kindness.

Working with Emotional Eating Regret

When you eat emotionally and feel regret afterward, it's easy to fall into harsh self-talk. But regret is not proof you did something "wrong"—it's an invitation to be curious, not cruel.

Instead of:
I shouldn't have eaten that.
Try:
I was doing the best I could in that moment. What was I feeling? What did I need? What other choices might be available next time?

Rework one of your less-than-compassionate responses to emotional eating:

Working with Big or Unfamiliar Emotions

Some emotions—like rage, grief, jealousy, or deep sadness—can feel unfamiliar or un-safe.

Instead of trying to fix or suppress them, self-compassion invites you to *sit beside them* like a steady companion.

Instead of:

I can't handle this.

Try:

This is a lot, and I'm still here.
This feeling won't last forever. I can breathe through this moment.

Rework one of your automatic responses to big emotions:

Working with Frustration About Where You Are

Healing is not linear. You will revisit the same lessons many times. Sometimes, it feels like you're not making progress—but that doesn't mean you've failed.

Instead of:

I should be further along.

Try:

Growth is happening, even if I can't see it right now.
Every time I come back to this work, I deepen my understanding.

Rework one of your reactions to frustration:

The Three-Step Self-Compassion Statement

This formula can help you create supportive internal dialogue in moments of struggle:

1. When I feel . . .

(name the emotion or situation)

2. I will remind myself . . .

(compassionate truth)

3. And I will offer myself . . .

(supportive action, perspective, or response)

Create your own three-part self-compassion statement:

Try It

Use the prompts below to create your own self-compassionate statements based on
situations in this chapter:

1. When I emotionally eat and feel regret, I will remind myself . . .
    (e.g., I was coping in the only way I knew how in that moment.)

2. When I feel overwhelmed by emotion, I will offer myself . . .
    (e.g., a deep breath, a hand on my heart, and the reminder that this too will pass.)

3. When I feel like I'm not making progress, I will remind myself . . .
    (e.g., healing isn't a straight line, and showing up again is a sign of strength.)

Ongoing Practice

Self-compassion isn't a one-time fix—it's a way of being. The more often you practice speaking to yourself with tenderness, the more natural it becomes. Eventually, it becomes your baseline.

Reflection:

What's one phrase I want to carry with me when things feel hard?

How will I practice offering that phrase in the moments I need it most?

Chapter 3 Key Takeaways

- Emotional work is essential for healing your relationship with food and body.
- Suppressing emotions often leads to unwanted eating patterns—not because you're weak, but because you're human.
- Your nervous system must feel safe to allow emotional awareness.
- Meeting basic biological needs creates the foundation for tolerating and understanding emotional experiences.
- Every emotion has something to teach you—none are wrong or shameful.
- Some emotions may be unfamiliar or uncomfortable, but they become more approachable with practice.
- Unprocessed trauma can complicate emotional work—discernment and pacing are acts of wisdom.
- All experiences—emotions, meals, cravings—follow a predictable arc: arising, peaking, dissolving.
- Practicing mindfulness helps shift unconscious neuroception into conscious interoception and insight.
- Zooming in (feeling) and zooming out (gaining perspective) are both necessary for emotional balance.
- Emotional eating is one valid coping strategy—what matters is having more than one option.
- Desires and "other hungers," like connection, pleasure, purpose, and expression, are real and worthy of attention.
- When deeper needs are unmet, turning to food makes sense—especially when food is one of the few safe, accessible sources of comfort.
- Self-compassion is not indulgent—it's foundational to healing, resilience, and sustained change.
- You can grow your emotional literacy with practice, curiosity, and care.

The Trunk: Satisfaction

With your foundational needs met, you can begin to connect with the experience of enough. The trunk of the tree represents satisfaction: enough chocolate, enough pleasure, enough quiet, enough nature, enough connection. When you are satisfied, you are free. You can return to your life without fixation, shame, or regret.

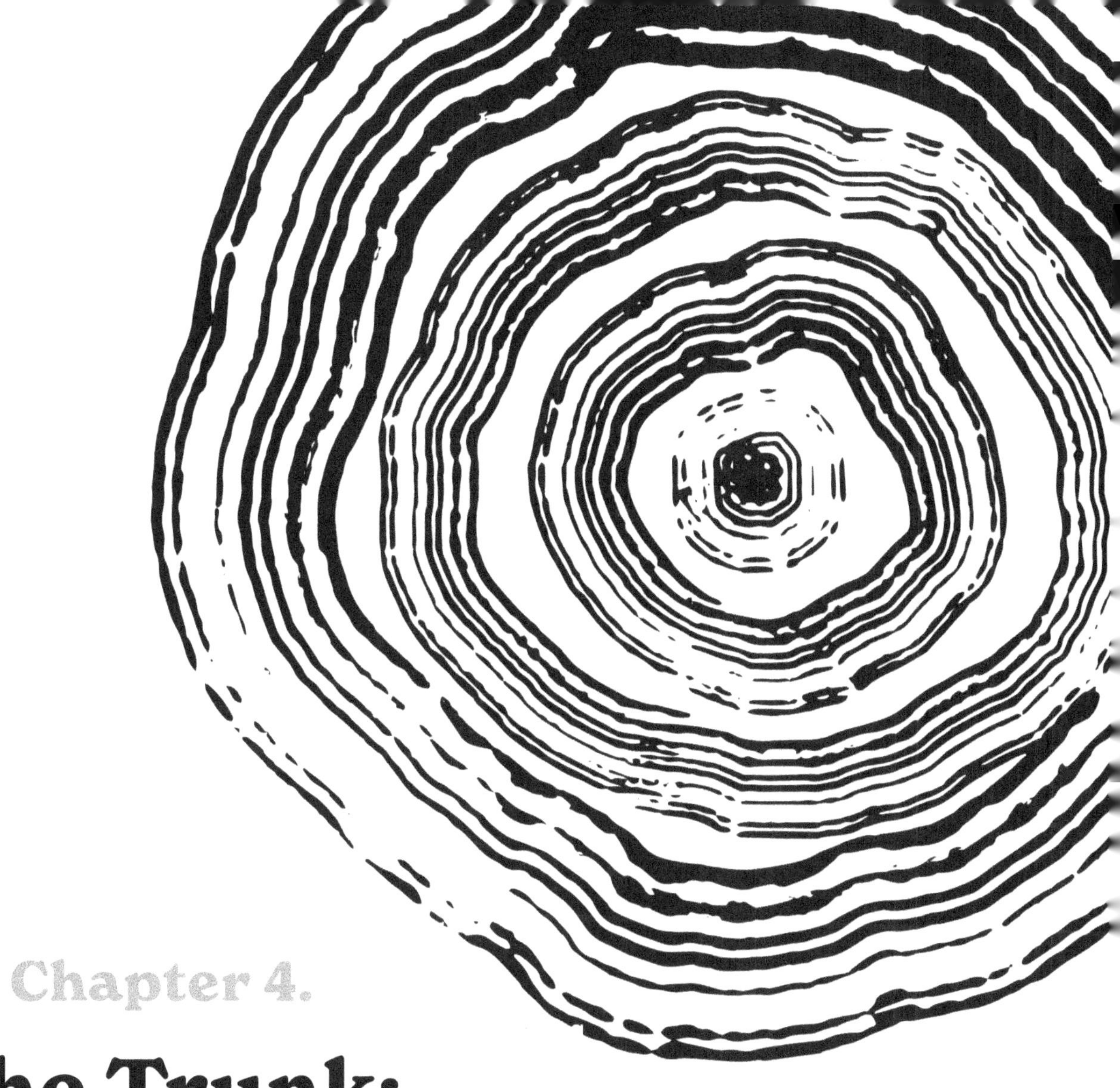

The Trunk: Satisfaction

The Paramitas (the how)

> *Generosity: I allow myself enough—nourishment, rest, connection, and gentleness.*

> *Discipline: I return to what's true, aligning action with respect.*

Patience: I honor slow growth and meet setbacks with compassion.

Exertion: I show up for myself with joyful, steady effort.

Meditation: I rest with what is, without fixing or fleeing.

> *Wisdom: I see clearly and act from clarity and compassion.*

Satisfaction: Why It Matters

In the Intuitive Eating Ecosystem, satisfaction is the radiant center of the mandala—a dynamic, living core that gives coherence and vitality to the entire process.

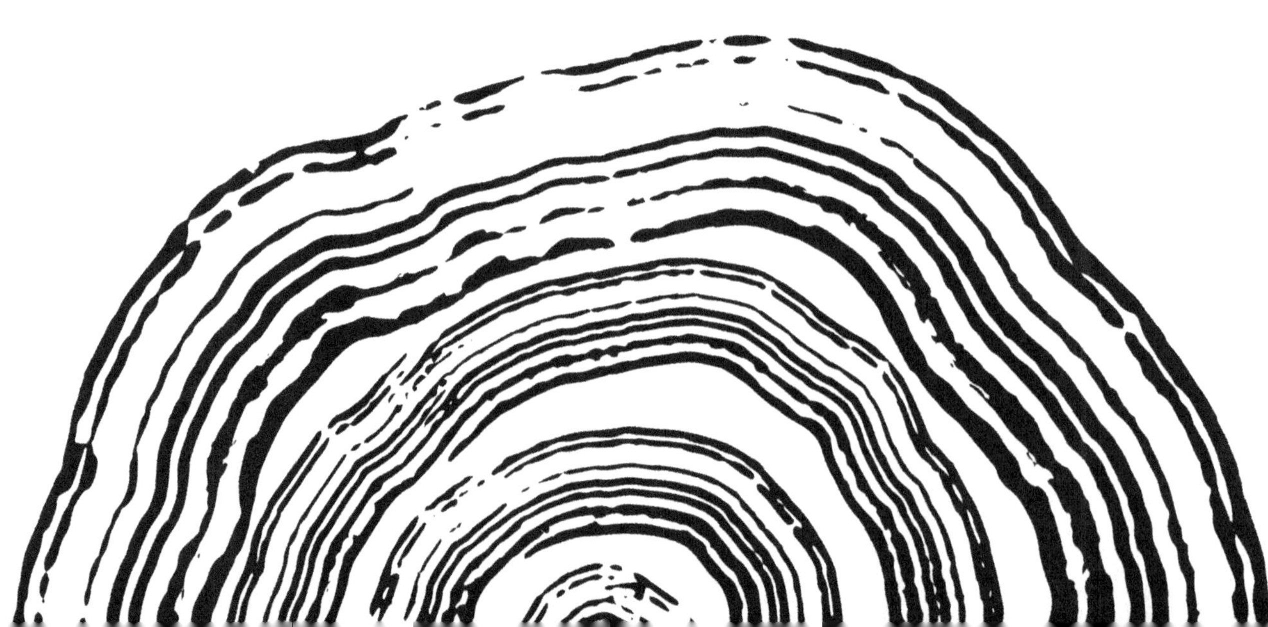

It is the point where body, mind, and heart converge. In Buddhist teachings, the center of the mandala represents wholeness and integration. Likewise, in mindful, Intuitive Eating, satisfaction brings together biological needs, emotional nourishment, and cognitive clarity into a single, grounded experience of enoughness.

Satisfaction is more than just a pleasant feeling; it is an embodied sense of having been tended to. It arises when your needs are recognized and honored, when eating is not just functional but pleasurable, and when your internal cues guide you without fear or conflict. In this way, satisfaction becomes both the goal and the method. The more you center satisfaction, the more peaceful and attuned your relationship with food becomes.

In this chapter, you will learn about the complex and essential nature of satisfaction. And you'll practice finding satisfaction in eating and elsewhere.

The Link Between Satisfaction and Interoception

To know what satisfies you, you must be able to feel it—in your body, your emotions, and your attention. This is the work of interoception: the internal awareness of bodily sensations like hunger, fullness, pleasure, and comfort. When interoception is strong, you can sense satisfaction as it arises and honor it as a signpost, not a luxury.

As you begin to tune into satisfaction, you may notice that it softens the emotional charge around eating. Foods that once felt "forbidden" or "dangerous" lose their hold. Rigid rules begin to loosen. You start to trust that eating for satisfaction does not mean losing control, but rather, regaining presence.

Satisfaction as a Measure of Enoughness

Satisfaction is how we know something has been completed, fulfilled, or tended to. It signals the end of a meal, the moment to rest, or the completion of an experience. When we learn to seek satisfaction in food and life, we begin to understand what "enough" feels like—not as a restriction, but as a grounded, nurturing boundary. This is especially important for those who have learned to override their needs in the name of productivity, control, or perfection.

Barriers to Satisfaction

Even though satisfaction is a natural part of being human, many of us have learned to distrust it. The pursuit of satisfaction is often seen as indulgent, selfish, or even dangerous. This conditioning starts early and is reinforced by diet culture, hustle culture, and moralized narratives around food and pleasure.

Common barriers include:
- Internalized guilt or shame around enjoying food
- Disconnection from hunger and fullness cues due to chronic dieting
- Beliefs that pleasure must be earned or justified
- Overriding the body's signals to meet external expectations
- Fear that satisfaction will lead to loss of control

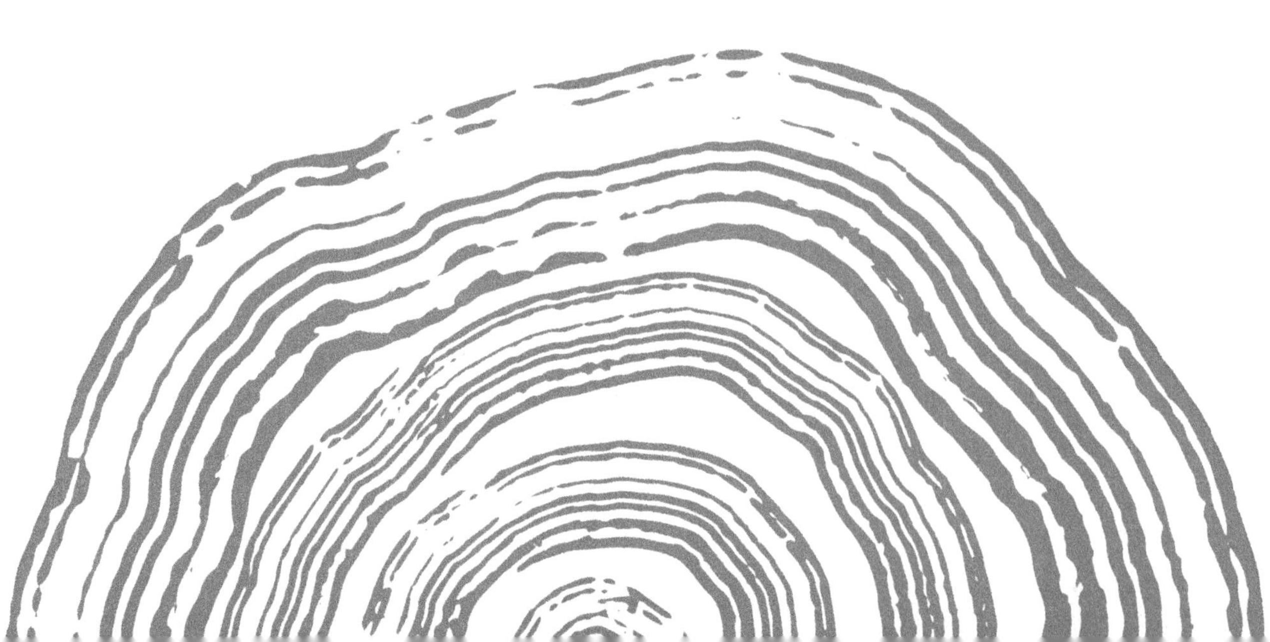

What messages have I received about satisfaction or pleasure?

When have I felt judged (by others or myself) for enjoying something fully?

How do these beliefs show up in my relationship with food today?

Discovering What Satisfies You

You can strengthen your connection to satisfaction by asking: What truly nourishes me? What delights me? What leaves me feeling grounded and whole?

Explore the following domains:

Food: What textures, flavors, temperatures, and combinations bring you joy? What leaves you feeling energized and content?

Clothing: What feels good on your skin? What helps you feel like yourself?

Temperatures: Do you feel best in warmth or coolness? How can you create comfort in your environment?

Relaxation: What kinds of rest restore you?

Fun: What kinds of play, laughter, or lightness bring you into the moment?

Curiosity: What engages your mind, inspires your thoughts, or draws you into flow?

Nature: What kind of natural environments feed your soul—water, trees, open skies?

Additional Noticings:

Practice: Cultivating Satisfaction Awareness

Each day, take a moment to reflect:

- What felt satisfying today?
- What was missing?
- Where did I override satisfaction in the name of "should" or expectations?
- How might I return to myself tomorrow?

Reflection:

Micro-Satisfactions: The Building Blocks of Pleasure

Satisfaction doesn't have to be grand or dramatic. In fact, micro-satisfactions—small moments of sensory or emotional pleasure—are often what stitch our days together with meaning and warmth.

Examples:

- The first sip of a warm beverage
- A moment of quiet before bed
- A deep breath with your hand on your heart
- The warmth of sunlight on your skin
- A song that hits just right

Tuning into micro-satisfactions helps train your nervous system to recognize that nourishment is already here, even in small ways. These moments matter.

Reflection:

What micro-satisfactions did you experience today?

How did you respond to them?

Mindfulness Exercises for Working with Satisfaction

1. **Satisfaction Scan:** At the end of each meal, pause and ask yourself: *Did that meal satisfy me? What aspects contributed to or detracted from satisfaction?* Track your experience over a week to identify patterns and preferences.

2. **Pleasure Pause:** In the middle of a meal, take one mindful bite. Close your eyes. What flavors, textures, temperatures do you notice? Are you still enjoying it, or is satisfaction beginning to fade?

3. **Interoceptive Journaling:** Before and after eating, note: *How hungry am I? How satisfied do I feel? How do I know?* Use body-based descriptions (e.g., warmth in the belly, calm in the chest) to deepen awareness.

4. **Micro-Satisfaction Tracker:** Choose three small moments each day to pause and reflect: *What tiny act of pleasure or comfort did I just experience?* Note it down, and describe how it felt in your body.

The Pleasure Permission Slip

Sometimes we need explicit permission to reclaim what's always been ours.

Your Permission Slip:

I, _________________, give myself full permission to enjoy _________________

without guilt, shame, or justification. My body deserves pleasure.

My joy is not a problem.

Signed, _________________.

Reflection:

What would it mean to give yourself full permission to enjoy eating? How might that change your day-to-day experience with food?

Journaling Prompts to Track Satisfaction

- What does satisfaction feel like in my body?
- When was the last time I felt deeply satisfied? What contributed to that feeling?
- Are there areas of my life where satisfaction is consistently missing?
- What small acts bring a sense of contentment?
- How has my relationship with satisfaction shifted since beginning this work?
- What micro-satisfactions can I prioritize each day?

Making Peace with Food Through Satisfaction

When satisfaction becomes a guiding principle, food loses its moral charge. You no longer need to earn your meals or prove your worth. You are allowed to enjoy what you eat. This simple shift changes everything: from frantic consumption to presence, from guilt to permission, from chaos to peace.

The more you listen for satisfaction, the more you align with your body's wisdom. And the more you honor satisfaction, the more fully you inhabit your life.

Chapter 4 Key Takeaways

- Satisfaction is central to Intuitive Eating—it integrates body, heart, and mind.
- Interoception helps you recognize satisfaction as a bodily and emotional signal.
- Satisfaction is not indulgent—it's a sign you've been tended to.
- Honoring satisfaction promotes peace with food and reduces reactive eating.
- Micro-satisfactions help build awareness of pleasure in everyday life.
- Barriers to satisfaction often come from cultural conditioning and a diet mentality.
- You can relearn what satisfies you through curiosity, mindfulness, and permission.
- Tracking satisfaction reveals patterns and increases trust in your preferences.
- Giving yourself permission to enjoy food is a radical act of self-respect.
- The more you prioritize satisfaction, the more attuned and peaceful your relationship with food becomes.

The Branches: Expansion

When peace with food is established, you naturally branch out into more advanced elements of Intuitive Eating: stopping when comfortably full; engaging in regular, joyful movement; integrating gentle nutrition based on what your body truly needs. These branches don't represent rules—they are expressions of trust, connection, and care. They are what grow when you nurture the whole tree.

The Branches: Expansion

The Paramitas (the how)

Generosity: I allow myself enough—nourishment, rest, connection, and gentleness.

Discipline: I return to what's true, aligning action with respect.

> *Patience: I honor slow growth and meet setbacks with compassion.*

> *Exertion: I show up for myself with joyful, steady effort.*

> *Meditation: I rest with what is, without fixing or fleeing.*

Wisdom: I see clearly and act from clarity and compassion.

Expanding Your Ecosystem

This chapter focuses on the longer-term, more complex aspects of Intuitive Eating—nutrition, movement, and fullness.

These are the "leaves and branches" of your Intuitive Eating Ecosystem, supported by the strong roots and vibrant center you've already cultivated, sustained through the ongoing cognitive and emotional work you've learned to practice. Just as trees take time to grow and reach their full expression, these areas require patience, compassion, and ongoing curiosity.

Many people feel pressure to address these topics first—but jumping in too soon can reinforce old patterns of perfectionism or self-judgment. If you're still working on foundation-building, emotional regulation, or satisfaction, it's okay to hold off. There's no rush. These practices will wait for you.

In this chapter, you will learn how to approach the expansion of your Intuitive Eating practice. You'll practice assessing readiness, accepting where you are, and progressing at the right pace for you.

Before diving into each of these areas, take a moment to reflect:

Readiness Reflections:

- Am I approaching this from a place of curiosity or self-criticism?
- Do I feel emotionally resourced enough to explore this right now?
- What would feel like a small, doable step forward?

Movement: Reclaiming Joy in Motion

Movement is not a punishment or obligation—it's a way of being in your body. But because it's been so closely tied to weight loss, productivity, and morality, movement can feel loaded or even triggering. Reclaiming it means approaching it gently, on your own terms.

At its core, the human body wants to move. Babies stretch, squirm, and reach with wonder. Animals shake, roll, leap, and rest without shame. This is movement radiating from within, not surveilled from the outside.

That's the movement we're returning to here—not the kind that says, *You should be doing more*, but the kind that asks, *What feels good? What does my body want today?*

There are many types of movement: functional, expressive, playful, restorative, vigorous. Different things suit different bodies, abilities, seasons, and preferences. Your job isn't to find the "best" one—it's to discover what's right for you, today.

Pleasure is a valid, even necessary, motivation for movement. When your body feels tended to and included—not bullied or coerced—movement becomes something you look forward to, not something you dread or avoid.

When You Might Be Ready:

- You feel curious or inspired to move without guilt or pressure.
- You want to build a new relationship with your body—one rooted in care rather than control.
- You've let go of exercising as punishment or penance.
- You're drawn to movement to improve flexibility, balance, or ease of motion in daily life.
- You'd like to build stamina or feel stronger in ways that support how you live.
- You're interested in how movement might help alleviate discomfort or pain.
- You miss the feeling of being alive, present, or expressive in your body.
- You feel ready to try something new, exhilarating, or playful—or to move in a new environment, like nature.
- You're noticing a spark of motivation that feels different—not from shame or pressure, but from a desire to be in connection with yourself.

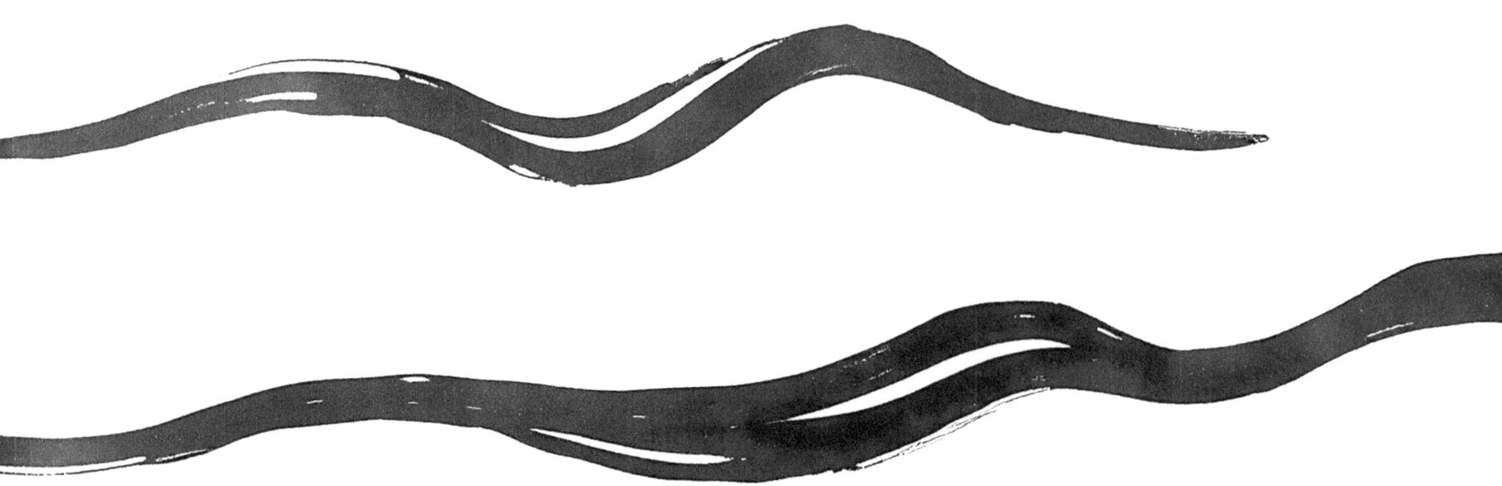

Reflection: What's Moving You?

Take a few moments to reflect on what's drawing you toward movement right now. There's no right or wrong answer—only useful information.

Which of the following motivations resonate with you today?

(Check any that apply—or write in your own.)

- ☐ I want to feel more connected to my body.

- ☐ I'm curious about what kinds of movement I might enjoy.

- ☐ I want to feel stronger or more capable.

- ☐ I'd like to ease some pain or physical discomfort.

- ☐ I miss the feeling of energy or aliveness in my body.

- ☐ I want to improve flexibility or fluidity.

- ☐ I'd like to build stamina or endurance.

- ☐ I want to experience joy, pleasure, or play.

- ☐ I want to be outside or connect with nature.

- ☐ I feel ready to try something new or exhilarating.

- ☐ I want to support my mental health.

- ☐ I'm looking for stress relief or emotional release.

- ☐ Other: _______________________________________

Which of these motivations feel nourishing and self-directed?

Are there any that feel tangled with old patterns of guilt,
shame, or obligation?

What's one small action I could take today that aligns with
a motivation I feel good about?

When You Might Want to Wait:

- You feel triggered by any mention of exercise.
- Movement still feels like a "should" more than a "want."
- You're using movement to earn food or shrink your body.
- You notice your mind tightening around movement—wanting to do more, go harder, or see results quickly.
- You feel guilt or shame when you miss a day of movement or don't push yourself hard enough.
- You find yourself dissociating from your body during movement or disconnecting from its cues.
- You compare your body harshly to others in motion.
- Your relationship with food and movement is getting tangled (e.g., restricting on rest days or eating based on exercise rather than hunger.)

Reflection: Honoring Where You Are With Movement

Before diving deeper into movement, take a moment to check in with your current experience:

What emotions arise when you think about exercise or physical activity?

Are there any "shoulds" or rules you notice creeping in?

Invitation: If this reflection reveals tension, grief, or ambivalence, that's not a failure—it's sacred information.

Gently consider:

What would feel like compassion, not compliance, in this moment?

Write down one act of kindness or curiosity you could offer your body today.

Ways to Begin:

- Try a short walk, and pay attention to sensations—not calories burned.
- Explore different movement intensities, durations, and preferences. Notice what feels best.
- Create a "movement menu"—activities you enjoy, from stretching to dancing to gardening.
- Experiment with low-pressure options like restorative yoga, swimming, tai chi, or mindful walking.
- Play with music—try moving to one song that lifts your mood.
- Get curious about motivation. Are you avoiding movement out of fatigue or disconnection—or is there something that might feel good?
- Reframe "laziness" as an opportunity to listen more deeply.
- Track how you feel *after* different kinds of movement, to identify patterns of enjoyment or nourishment.

Reflection:

What type of movement feels good today? What might my body be asking for?

Reflection During Movement:
What Keeps You Coming Back?

As you move, gently tune into your inner experience. Not every session will feel magical, but even small glimmers of connection can keep your practice alive.

See if any of these resonate as you reflect in the moment:

1. I want to reconnect with my body.

2. Look what my body can do!

3. This feels so good.

4. This is what my body is asking for.

You might also notice something else entirely. Let that awareness guide you. Returning to these doorways can help you stay grounded in joy and embodiment, rather than pressure or perfectionism.

Movement Reflection: After Moving

Which doorway did I pass through today (if any)?

What sensations, emotions, or thoughts arose during movement?

Did anything surprise me or feel different from what I expected?

What did this experience teach me about what my body needs—
or doesn't need—right now?

Is there anything I'd like to try again, adjust, or explore next time?

Adjusting Your Movement Practice

Bodies change. Life changes. What once felt good or easy might not anymore—and that doesn't mean you're failing. It just means it's time to adjust. Compassionate flexibility is key to maintaining a sustainable, joyful movement practice over the long term.

There are many reasons why your movement practice might need to shift:

- Weather or seasonal changes that affect your access or preferences.
- Gyms, classes, or communities becoming unavailable or changing.
- Injury or illness that changes what's possible or safe.
- Changes in routine—parenting demands, caregiving, travel, work stress.
- Shifting desires or preferences—what felt great once might not now.
- Evolving body needs—menstruation, perimenopause, chronic conditions, recovery.
- Mental or emotional shifts—sometimes, rest or stillness is the movement we need most.

Adjustments are not detours—they're part of the path, and a way to make your relationship with movement a lifelong thing. Listening, responding, and adapting are signs of a deepening relationship with your body.

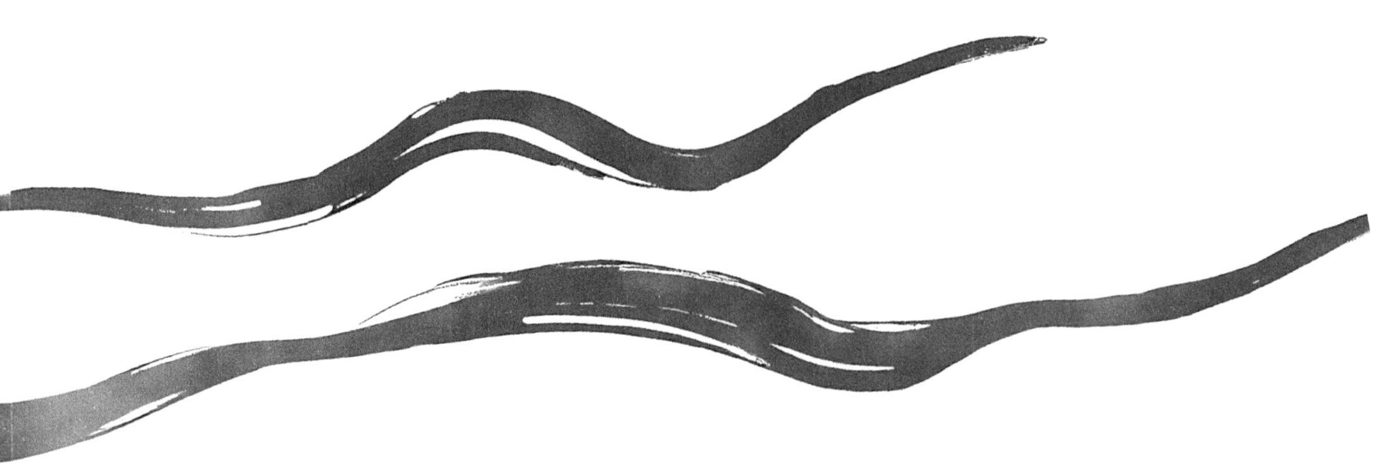

Reflection: Honoring What's Changing

What has changed in my life or body recently that might affect how I move?

Am I allowing my movement practice to evolve—or trying to force it
to stay the same?

What's something small I could try that fits my current needs?

Can I trust that changing my routine doesn't mean giving up—
that it might be a deeper act of self-care?

Nutrition: Gentle, Curious, Flexible

Nutrition is important—but it doesn't need to be rigid or punitive. In Intuitive Eating, we refer to this as *gentle nutrition,* because it respects both the science of nourishment and your lived experience of food. It's about patterns and practice, not perfection.

Approaching nutrition consciously and with compassion is essential. The way we feed ourselves is shaped by so many factors—our biology, our history, our current access and capacity. Working with nutrition isn't about fixing yourself or avoiding future pain. It's about supporting your body from a place of care, not fear.

This process requires patience and a tolerance for uncertainty. Despite what wellness culture might promise, eating a certain way is not a guarantee of perfect health. If health takes a turn, that doesn't mean you failed. It means you're human. Nourishment is about doing the best you can with what you know and what you're capable of in any given moment.

And like all things in this practice, it's a process of refinement. You try something, notice how it feels, and adjust. You return to curiosity instead of perfectionism. Because this isn't about getting it "right." It's about supporting yourself in a way that feels doable, kind, and nourishing.

When You Might Be Ready:

- You're mostly free from a diet mentality.
- You're eating consistently and honoring hunger.
- You want to feel better, not control your body.
- You suspect certain foods may be affecting your well-being and want to explore that with curiosity.
- You're interested in improving the overall nutritional quality of your meals—not perfectly, just gently.
- You're feeling drawn to add more variety to what you eat: colors, textures, flavors, densities.
- You want to support your body through a specific medical condition or life chapter.

- You're eating to support an athletic pursuit or to feel more energized for daily movement.
- You're ready to care for your body with more precision, not restriction.

Reflection: What's Drawing You Toward Nutrition?

What are some signs that you might be ready to explore gentle nutrition?

What hopes, fears, or intentions do you notice?

How might you bring curiosity and kindness to this process?

When You Might Want to Wait:

- You still view food in moral terms (good/bad).
- You feel overwhelmed by nutrition information.
- You're using nutritional changes to try to control weight.
- Your interest in nutrition is tied to a reactive life event (e.g., a friend starting GLP-1 meds, a breakup, an upcoming vacation, a new medical diagnosis).
- You're trying to ease anxiety or uncertainty by "fixing" food instead of feeling what's underneath.
- You feel pressure to prove something to yourself or others through your eating habits.
- You're feeling disconnected from your body's cues and rhythms.
- You're approaching food from fear, not care.

Reflection: What's Fueling My Focus on Nutrition?

What's prompting my interest in nutrition right now?

Does it feel rooted in self-care or in control, comparison, or urgency?

If I slowed down, what might I notice about what I truly need?

Ways to Begin:
Nourishment Through Gentle Exploration

- Add, don't subtract. Start by incorporating more fiber, protein, or color on your plate. This sends a signal to your body that nourishment—not deprivation—is your goal.
- Learn the basics:
  - **Carbohydrates** (e.g., oats, rice, fruit, sweet potatoes): Provide quick energy.
  - **Proteins** (e.g., eggs, tofu, chicken, beans, yogurt): Support satiety and muscle repair.
  - **Fats** (e.g., olive oil, nuts, avocado, seeds): Help food feel satisfying and support brain health.
  - **Fiber** (e.g., whole grains, lentils, vegetables, berries): Supports digestion and blood sugar stability.

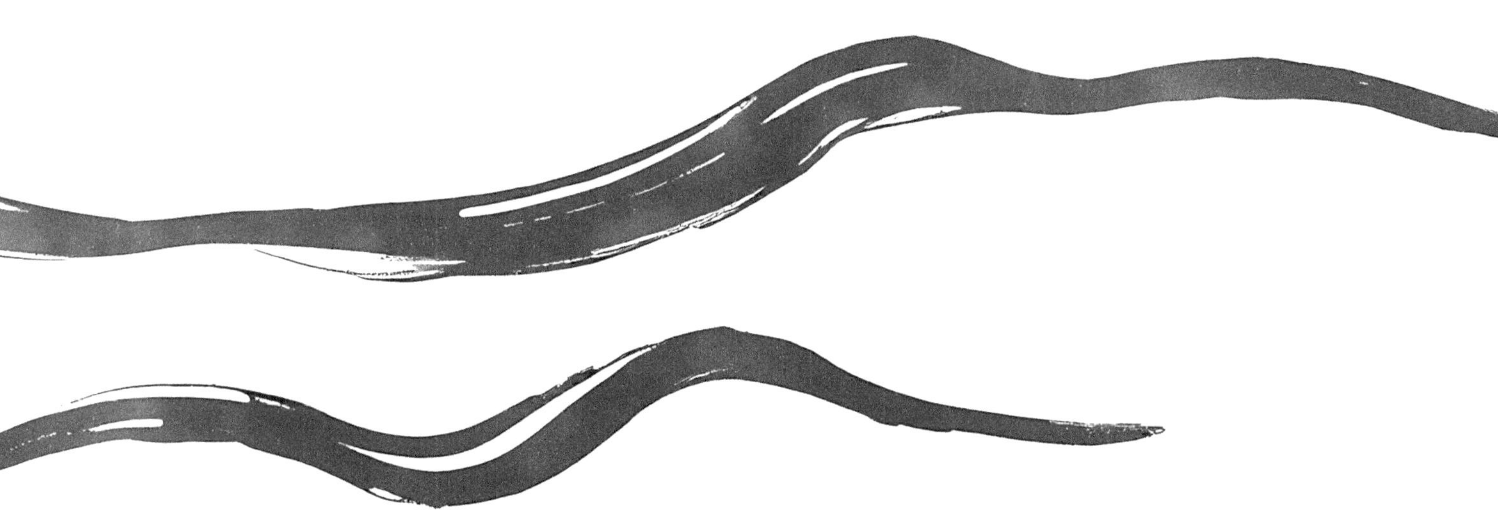

Meal and Snack Builder

Try combining at least two to three of the above components for more satisfaction and staying power. Use the table below for ideas, and create your own!

Meal/Snack	Carb	Protein	Fat	Fiber	Notes on How It Felt
Example: **Breakfast bowl**	*Oats*	*Greek yogurt*	*Peanut butter*	*Berries*	*Kept me full until lunch, felt warm and comforting*

Nourishment Tracking Reflection:

- How is my energy? (sluggish, steady, jittery)
- How does my mood feel?
- Any digestive reactions?
- Did this meal satisfy me—emotionally or physically?

What kind of nourishment helps me feel grounded, energized, or supported?

Adjusting With Life: Flexibility Over Perfection

The only constant in life—and in nourishment—is change.

Your nutrition needs will shift. The goal of Intuitive Eating is not to find a single approach that "works" and then cling to it forever. Instead, it's to remain responsive to the ever-changing nature of your body, mind, and life circumstances.

You might find yourself needing to adjust how you eat because of:

- Changes in age, hormones, or life stage
- Injury, illness, or recovery from a medical condition
- Travel or disrupted routines
- Mental health challenges
- Evolving preferences and values
- Shifts in appetite, tolerances, or digestive patterns
- Seasonal rhythms or cultural cycles

None of this is a failure. It's just life. The more you can meet these moments with curiosity rather than rigidity, the more resilient and attuned your relationship with food will become.

Reflection: Adjusting with Compassion

Take some time to reflect on what's changing—and how you might adapt with care.

What's shifted recently in my body, mind, or life?

What feelings come up around this change?
Can I make space for them?

What kind of nourishment feels supportive now?

Is there anyone I can reach out to for support?

What gentle adjustment would help me feel more grounded?

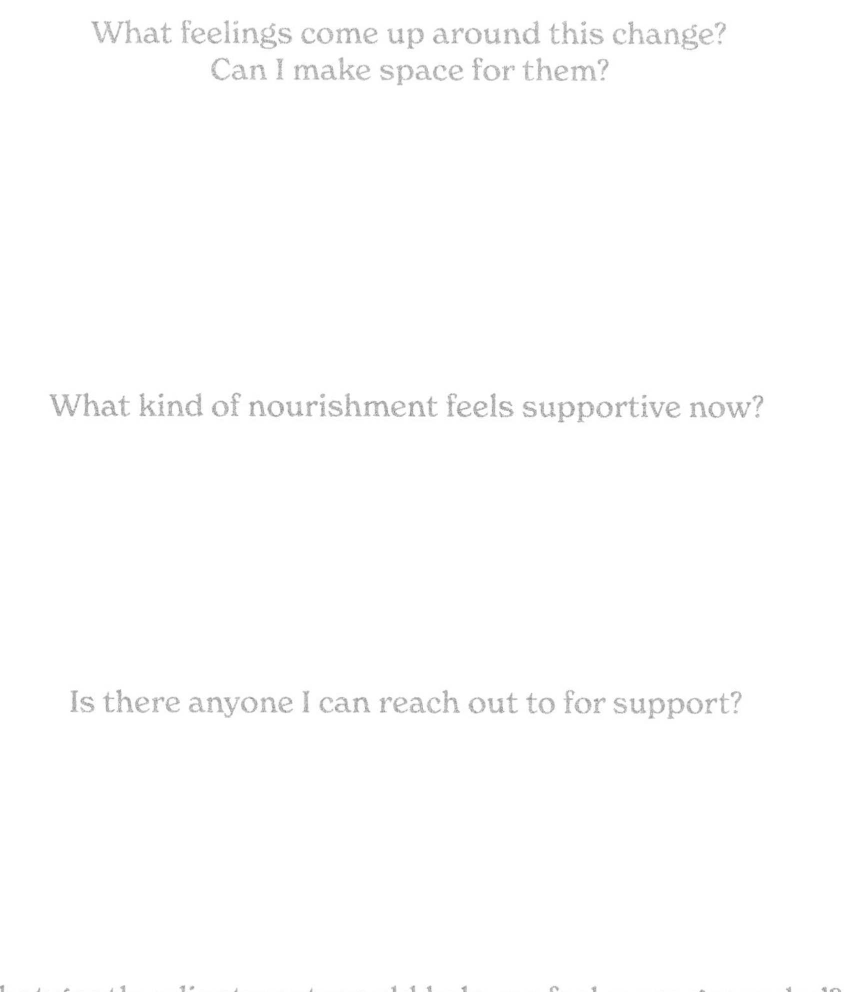

Fullness: Feeling into Enough

Honoring fullness can be incredibly healing—but also deeply complicated, especially if you've been taught to override or ignore it.

Many people come to Intuitive Eating convinced they eat "too much," so they want to focus on fullness right away. But if your body still believes deprivation is around the corner, trying to stop when you're comfortably full can feel like punishment—not self-care.

That's why fullness is a *later-stage* practice. In early healing, you need generosity. You need to convince your body it's safe—that food won't be withheld, that hunger isn't dangerous, and that satisfaction matters. Rushing into fullness cues too soon can activate old restriction-based behaviors, confuse your nervous system, and reignite shame.

Fullness isn't a moral checkpoint. It's a felt sense. And sometimes, that sense is hard to access—especially if you've been disconnected from your body, lived through food insecurity, experienced trauma, or internalized rigid rules around eating.

Here, we begin to reapproach fullness with gentleness and curiosity. You'll learn to feel into *your* "enough"—not based on a portion size or an external rule, but on interoception, trust, and embodied presence.

When You Might Be Ready:

- You feel safe responding to hunger and are eating consistently throughout the day.
- You're mostly free from extreme restriction or binging.
- You're curious about how your body communicates satisfaction and satiety.
- You notice a tendency to eat past comfortable fullness in a way that reduces your satisfaction.
- You want to explore the early, subtle cues of fullness—before discomfort or guilt sets in.
- You're beginning to trust that stopping at comfortable fullness doesn't make you "good" or "bad."
- You feel ready to stay with your own "edge"—the growing place where discomfort and curiosity meet.

Reflection: Approaching Fullness with Curiosity

What happens—physically, emotionally, or mentally—when you begin to feel full?

Have you ever noticed a shift in satisfaction when you eat past the point of fullness?

What's your relationship to stopping? Does it feel like care, control, or something else?

How might it feel to explore the edges of fullness without judgment?

Are you willing to trust that comfort and adequacy—not restriction—can guide you?

When You Might Want to Wait:

- You often eat past fullness out of fear you won't get more.
- You're still healing from deprivation or scarcity.
- You associate fullness with failure or loss of control.
- You feel guilt or shame when you eat past comfortable fullness.
- You notice yourself eating in response to discomfort or pain, especially in reactive or automatic ways.
- You find that focusing on fullness is making your thinking more rigid or rule-based.
- You're using fullness cues as a proxy for morality—feeling "bad" for not stopping at the "right" moment.
- You feel anxious or preoccupied with trying to "get it right."

Reflection: Honoring the Complexity of Fullness

What stories or beliefs do I hold about fullness?

When I eat past fullness, how do I interpret that moment?

What feelings come up when I try to stop at comfortable fullness?

Am I using fullness as a measurement of success—or as a signal of care?

What would it feel like to trust that I can stay curious,
even when things feel messy?

Ways to Begin:

- **Practice Pausing Mid-Meal:**

  Halfway through eating, gently pause—not to judge, but to notice. How's your pace? Are you still enjoying it? What's your current level of fullness?

- **Use a Fullness Scale:**

  Try rating your fullness on a 1–10 scale (1 = ravenous, 10 = painfully full). What does a 6 feel like? An 8? Track how your body feels at different points.

- **Distinguish Between Fullness and Satisfaction:**

  You might feel physically full but still unsatisfied—or satisfied with a smaller portion. Both types of feedback matter. Notice how fullness and satisfaction interact.

- **Journal the Context:**

  Reflect on how fullness feels in different settings:
  - Alone vs. with others
  - At home vs. out at a restaurant
  - During calm vs. stress
  - With familiar vs. new foods

- **Tune Into the Arc of Fullness:**

  After a meal, set a timer for thirty to sixty minutes. Revisit your sensations. Do you feel content, sluggish, still hungry? Use this data as part of your self-knowledge, not judgment.

Reflection:

What does fullness feel like in my body right now?

Are there early cues I've been missing?

What's my tendency—do I usually stop too early, or go past my edge?

How does emotional context (stress, joy, loneliness)
influence my experience of fullness?

How would I describe "enough" in my own words—not someone else's?

Deepening as a Lifelong Practice

There's no finish line in Intuitive Eating—only a deeper spiral into self-awareness, trust, and compassion. As your life changes, so will your body, preferences, needs, and capacities. That's not a problem—it's the nature of being alive.

This chapter is about allowing complexity and practicing responsiveness. Nutrition, movement, and fullness are rich, layered topics that deserve your patience. You don't need to "get them right" once and for all. You only need to keep listening and adjusting.

Progress in this work isn't linear. You'll revisit old patterns, uncover new insights, and circle back to foundational practices again and again. That's not backsliding—it's integration.

Keep checking in. Keep offering yourself care. Keep returning to the roots: nourishment, connection, satisfaction, and compassion. You're already in the process.

Ongoing Reflections:

- Am I approaching this with gentleness or pressure?
- What support might I need right now?
- What's one small step that honors my current capacity?
- What do I want to revisit from earlier chapters?
- Where am I noticing growth?

Chapter 5 Key Takeaways

- Intuitive Eating is a lifelong practice, not a linear path or destination.
- Movement, nutrition, and fullness are nuanced areas best approached with curiosity, not pressure.
- Readiness is key—there's no shame in waiting until the time feels right.
- Sustainable change grows from self-knowledge, not guilt or obligation.
- Movement can be joyful, adaptive, and rooted in inner desire—not external expectations.
- Gentle nutrition honors science and lived experience, with room for flexibility and pleasure.
- Fullness is deeply individual and can shift based on context, emotion, and history.
- Adjustments are a natural and necessary part of long-term care. Nothing is fixed forever.
- Returning to the foundations—emotional awareness, satisfaction, and compassion—will always serve you.

The Air: Trauma-Informed Mindfulness

Air is the spaciousness of presence. It reminds us to work gently with our nervous systems, to engage mindfully with life as it unfolds. Mindfulness might look like meditation, breathwork, a body scan, or a simple check-in. The key is discernment: learning to sense when to lean into discomfort—and when to step back and return later. This is the practice of honoring your window of tolerance.

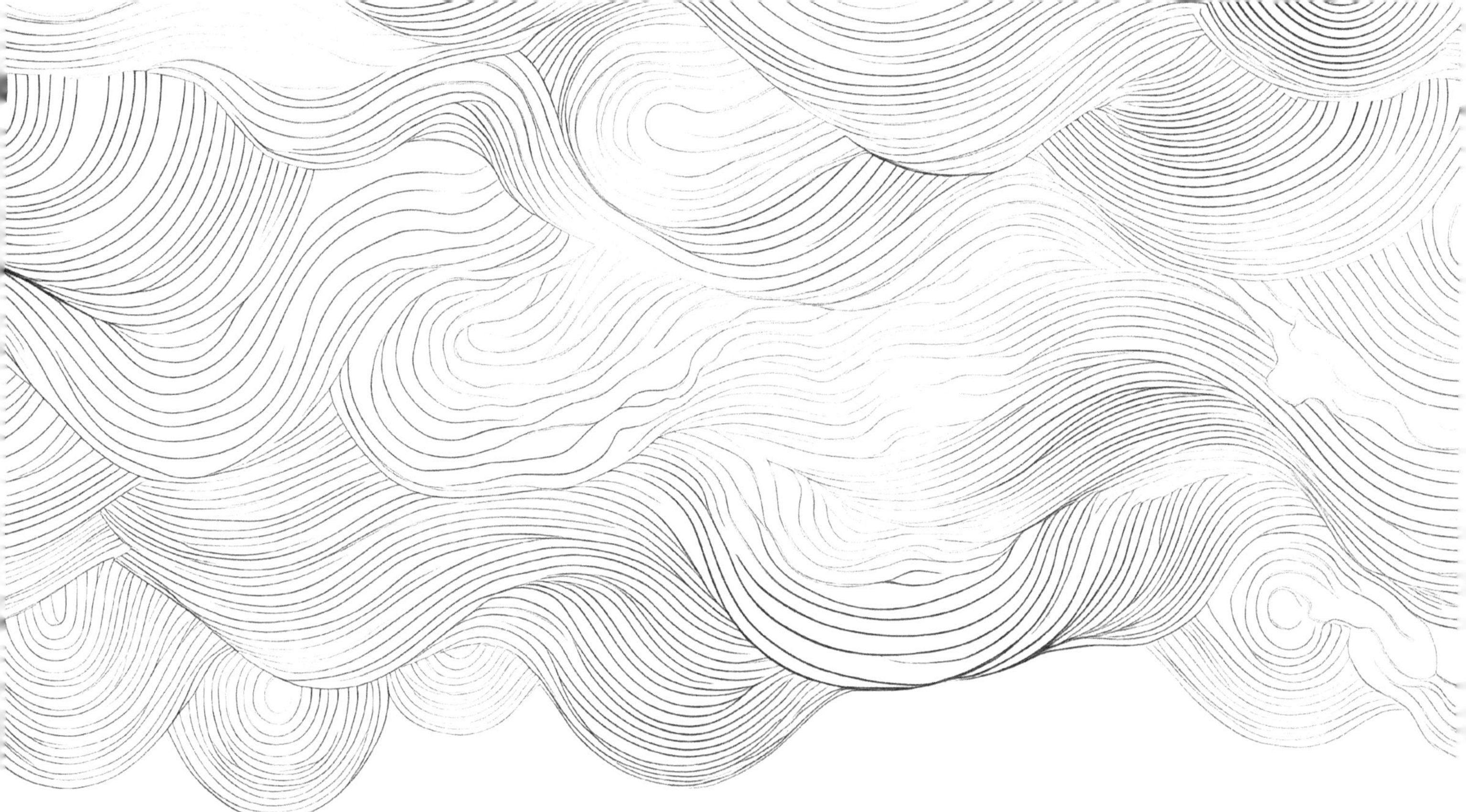

The Air:
Trauma-Informed Mindfulness

The Paramitas (the how)

> **Generosity:** *I allow myself enough—nourishment, rest, connection, and gentleness.*

Discipline: I return to what's true, aligning action with respect.

Patience: I honor slow growth and meet setbacks with compassion.

Exertion: I show up for myself with joyful, steady effort.

> **Meditation:** *I rest with what is, without fixing or fleeing.*

> **Wisdom:** *I see clearly and act from clarity and compassion.*

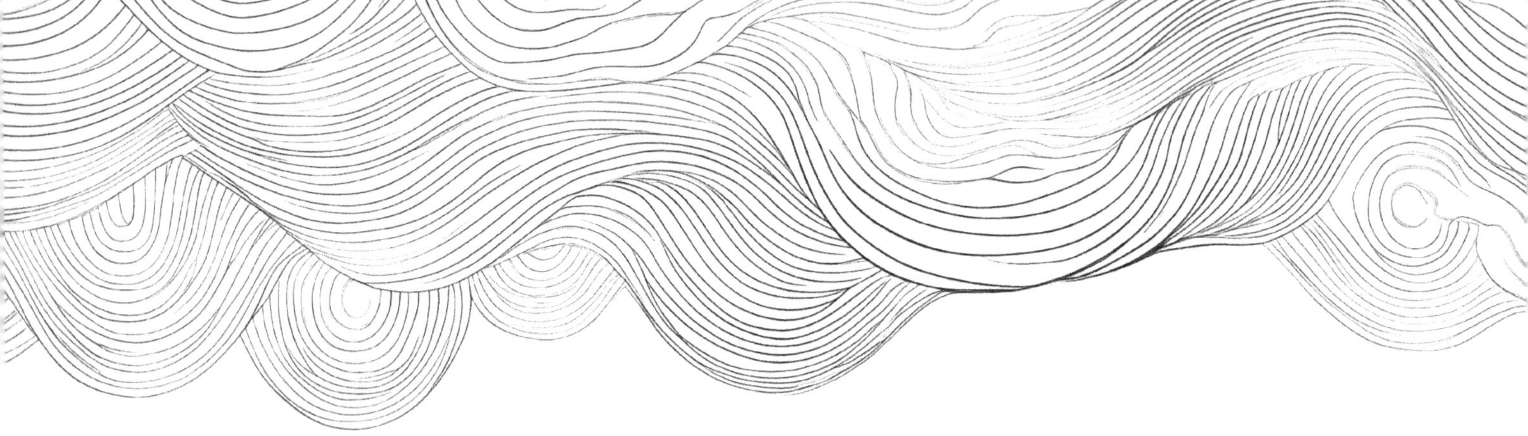

Walking the Path,
Over and Over Again

This final chapter is not about reaching an endpoint—it's about embracing Intuitive Eating as a lifelong path.

The journey is cyclical, full of change, growth, rest, and renewal. It's not always linear or clear, but it becomes more grounded as you develop a deeper sense of trust—in your body, your emotions, and your values.

To walk this path requires a particular view: one rooted in curiosity, compassion, and the recognition that obstacles are part of the path—not signs you've failed. In fact, each challenge is a teacher, pointing you back to your inner wisdom. You'll develop a somatic and emotional "knowing," a language for your body's cues, and the capacity to stay present with whatever arises.

You'll need patience, presence, gentleness, humor, connection, trust, and the ability to work with uncertainty. One of the most essential qualities on this path is equanimity.

Equanimity is often misunderstood. It doesn't mean being detached or emotionless—that's actually a form of spiritual bypassing. True equanimity is about staying connected to yourself even in the midst of emotional intensity. It means feeling your feelings fully without abandoning yourself, without needing to fix, escape, or suppress. It's the ability to hold joy, grief, fear, and confusion with the same open-hearted awareness.

This chapter will help you to understand various mindfulness practices and to choose which one is appropriate for you as your Intuitive Eating practice—and you!—evolve.

The Unfolding: Getting Comfortable in the Unknown

Growth often happens below the surface. Like crocuses peeking out after winter, your process may be invisible until suddenly, it emerges. Dormancy is not failure—it's ripening. This invisible labor—the softening, the reorienting, the preparation—can be hard to trust. But just as seeds require darkness, time, and nourishment before they bloom, your inner work also needs space to develop quietly.

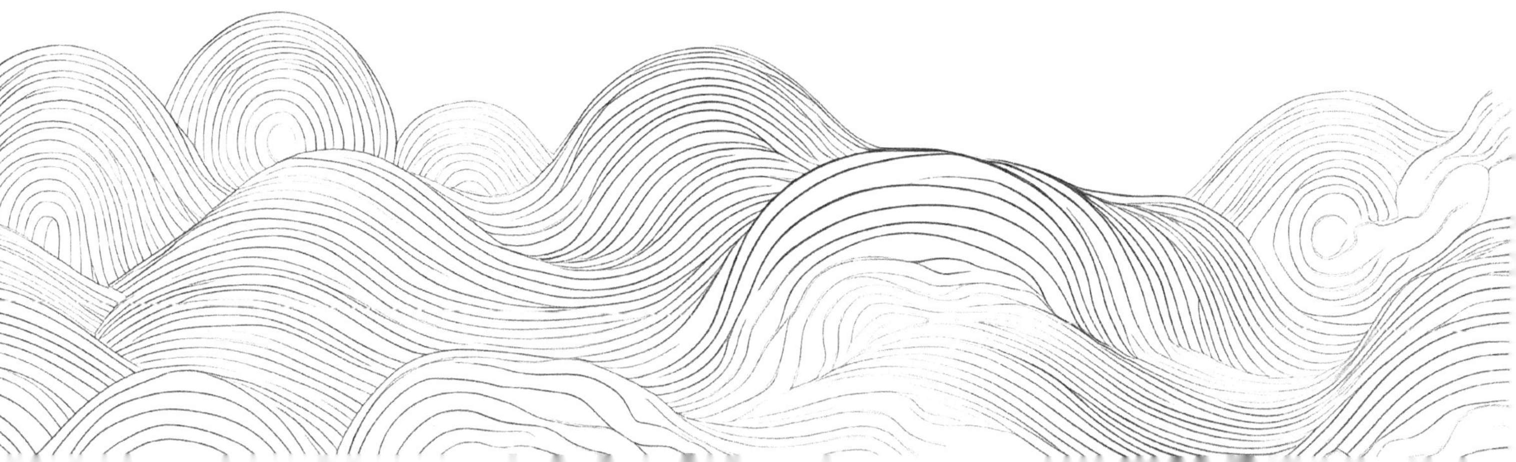

Reflection: Trusting Dormancy—Past and Present

Think of a time when you felt stuck, stalled, or convinced that progress had stopped. What was happening below the surface that you couldn't see at the time? How did things eventually shift?

Now, bring awareness to a current area of your life that feels dormant or uncertain. What might be quietly ripening or preparing to emerge? What would it feel like to trust the timing of your own unfolding?

Mantras for When You Feel Stalled:

- I trust in the unseen parts of my growth.
- This is part of the process.
- True healing takes time and patience.
- My inner work is still unfolding, even when I can't see it.
- I am growing in ways I don't yet understand.

My mantra:

Mantras for When It Feels Like You're Going Backwards:

- I haven't failed—I'm being asked to listen more deeply.
- I can begin again, as many times as I need to.
- This is a moment of stress, not a reversal.
- Old patterns feel familiar, but I am not the same person.
- Every step forward includes moments of return and review.

My mantra:

Meditation as Ongoing Support

Meditation is not about becoming someone different—it's about becoming *more yourself.* It's the practice of feeling: being with each breath as it comes and goes, allowing your body, your breath, your thoughts, and your emotions to be just as they are. It's about presence, not perfection.

Meditation helps you develop an expansive, embodied awareness—a way of being with yourself that includes all your emotional states, from ease to chaos. You learn to stay present when you feel joy, fear, grief, or frustration, and to greet those states with compassion rather than judgment. You begin to trust your capacity to feel deeply *without abandoning yourself.*

Meditation also trains you to observe the shifting landscape of your nervous system: the way your energy, moods, and sensations ebb and flow. None of it is permanent, and all of it is workable. This steadiness and perspective are invaluable as you deepen your relationship with food, body, and self.

The practice of *shamatha-vipashyana*—calm abiding and insight—is a foundational support for Intuitive Eating, allowing you to both settle the mind and clearly observe your inner experience.

Shamatha-Vipashyana Instructions:

1. Sit comfortably, spine upright but relaxed.
2. Place hands on thighs, palms facing down.
3. Gaze softly downward.
4. Bring attention to your breath—natural, unforced—and feel the sensation.
5. Allow thoughts to be as they are, and to come and go on their own.
6. When the mind wanders (and it will), gently label the thought "thinking" and return to the breath.
7. You get infinite opportunities to start fresh.

Posture Troubleshooting:

- Back pain? Try a cushion or chair with support.
- Hip pain? Try raising your seat a bit higher so the knees are lower than the hips.
- Fidgety? Place a bit more emphasis on the out breath, or shorten your sessions.
- Sleepy? Try meditating earlier in the day, or placing a bit more emphasis on the in breath.

Build Your Meditation Practice

On what days will I sit?	When during the day will I sit?
Where will I practice?	How long can I realistically sit?

What helps me re-enter after I fall out of the routine?

How can I track what I notice—mood, presence, insight?

Sustainability Tips:

- Keep it simple.
- Build routine through anchoring (same chair, time, journal).
- Expect the ups and downs.
- Use gentle re-entry phrases like: *Today is a good day to return.*

Trauma-Informed Mindfulness

Meditation can be a powerful support on the Intuitive Eating path—but it is not neutral. For trauma survivors, mindfulness may bring moments of deep healing *and* moments of overwhelm. This doesn't mean you're doing it wrong. It means your nervous system is working hard to protect you, and that needs to be honored.

Key Distinctions:

- Feeling uncomfortable but safe is part of growth. It may include restlessness, distraction, or even tears. These are not red flags—they are signs that you're beginning to feel and notice.
- Feeling unsafe, re-traumatized, dissociated, or panicked is different. This is your nervous system letting you know that something is too much, too fast. The wisest action may be to pause, shift practices, or seek support.

Mindfulness is not a one-size-fits-all practice. True trauma-sensitive mindfulness involves choice, agency, and gentleness at every step.

Signs to Pause or Modify Your Practice:

- Sudden numbness or a sense of "leaving" the body
- Flashbacks or intrusive thoughts
- Overwhelm that doesn't lessen with time
- A sense of being frozen or paralyzed

These are not failures. They're invitations to adjust your approach so it better supports your healing.

Supportive practices that may feel safer include:

- Grounding through the senses: name five things you see, four things you hear, three things you can touch, two things you can smell, one thing you can taste
- Gentle movement practices: walking meditation, stretching, rocking
- Support anchors: place one hand on your chest or belly, use weighted blankets, or hold an object
- Shorter practices: one- to three-minute check-ins instead of twenty-minute sits
- Eyes open or a soft gaze rather than closing the eyes
- Working with a trauma-informed teacher or therapist to co-create a safe practice container

Reflection:

What helps me feel grounded and safe when I feel activated or overwhelmed? How can I bring more of that into my mindfulness or self-care practice?

Additional Supportive Practices

As your relationship with food and body deepens, it can be helpful to draw on other meditative practices that cultivate warmth, compassion, and connection—especially when things feel stuck or overwhelming. The following practices can be layered gently into your routine. Each one begins with about five minutes of *shamatha* (calm abiding) to settle your mind and body and ends with another five minutes to return and integrate.

Lovingkindness Meditation (Metta)

Begin by sitting quietly and practicing *shamatha* for five minutes—just being with your breath. Then, bring yourself to mind and silently offer these phrases:

- May I be safe.
- May I be well.
- May I be free from suffering.
- May I live with ease.

Let each phrase drop in like a pebble into a pond. You don't have to force yourself to feel anything—just offer the words and notice what arises. After spending time with yourself, you might choose to offer these same phrases to someone you love, a neutral person, a difficult person, and eventually, to all beings.

Finish with five minutes of *shamatha* to settle and absorb.

Lovingkindness for the Body

Start with five minutes of breath awareness. Then, slowly bring attention to each part of your body, offering gratitude and care.

Thank you, feet, for carrying me.

Thank you, belly, for digesting my food.

There's no rush. You can do a full body scan or focus on just a few areas that need love today.

Close with five minutes of *shamatha* to rest in presence.

Tonglen Practice

After settling into your breath for five minutes, bring to mind a moment of discomfort—yours or someone else's. As you inhale, imagine breathing in the pain or suffering. As you exhale, offer compassion, ease, or relief.

Inhale: discomfort

Exhale: relief and compassion

This isn't about taking on others' suffering—it's about softening your resistance and opening the heart. Practice for a few minutes, then return to *shamatha* for integration.

Compassionate Body Scan

Begin with five minutes of *shamatha*. Then gently move your attention through the body—feet to head or head to feet—pausing with curiosity and care in each area.

You might think or whisper, *Hello, shoulders. You're holding so much. Thank you.*

If you encounter tension, numbness, or pain, see if you can greet it with kindness instead of judgment.

End with five minutes of *shamatha*, resting in the awareness you've cultivated.

Which did you try? What did you discover?

Chapter 6 Key Takeaways

- This is a lifelong, spiraling path—not a finish line.
- Your relationship with food and body will keep evolving.
- Obstacles and setbacks are invitations, not failures.
- Growth often happens below the surface—trust the unseen.
- Dormancy is not stagnation; it's ripening.
- You already have what you need to keep going.
- Meditation builds your capacity to feel, observe, and stay.
- Equanimity means feeling everything without self-abandonment.
- True mindfulness honors your nervous system's needs.
- There is no one right way—your path is your own.
- Begin again, gently, as often as you need to.
- Let presence, humor, and compassion lead the way.

A Final Word

This workbook isn't perfect—because perfection was never the point. What it *is*, I hope, is a powerful collection of tools, practices, and reflections to help you know yourself more deeply, more compassionately, and more honestly.

You can return to these pages anytime. Let them meet you where you are. As you grow, so too will your relationship with Intuitive Eating, mindfulness, and the beautiful, complicated body you live in. There's no final destination—only deepening, remembering, and beginning again.

If this work has supported you, inspired a shift, or stirred something new, I would be honored to hear about it. And if something didn't land quite right, I welcome that, too. You can reach me at jenna@jennahollenstein.com—I'd love to hear your celebrations or reflections.

Thank you for bringing your full, messy, magnificent self to this path. Keep going. Keep listening. You're doing beautifully.

With love,
Jenna

Additional Worksheets

Worksheet: Structured Eating Plans

Example: **Structured eating plan #1** **Structured eating plan #2**

[6:00 am] Wake

[7:00 am] Breakfast

[10:00 am] Snack

[1:00 pm] Lunch

[4:00 pm] Snack

[7:00 pm] Dinner

[10:00 pm] Snack

[10:30 pm] Bed

Structured eating plan #3 **Structured eating plan #4** **Structured eating plan #5**

Worksheet: Personal Hunger Scale

Fill in the scale below to better clarify what hunger feels like in *your* body:

1____

2____

3____

4____

5____

6____

7____

8____

9____

10____

What do you notice about the progression of hunger in your body?

What do you notice about the connection between hunger level and pleasure while eating?

At what hunger level do you enjoy food the most?

At what level of hunger do you tend to start eating, and how does that affect your eating experience?

Worksheet: Thought Reframing Practice

Original thought: ____

What makes this thought feel true: _______________________________________

A more flexible, truthful reframe: _______________________________________

____

How does this new thought feel in your body? _______________________________

Original thought: ____

What makes this thought feel true: _______________________________________

A more flexible, truthful reframe: _______________________________________

____

How does this new thought feel in your body? _______________________________

Original thought: ____

What makes this thought feel true: ____

A more flexible, truthful reframe: ____

____

How does this new thought feel in your body? ____

Original thought: ____

What makes this thought feel true: ____

A more flexible, truthful reframe: ____

____

How does this new thought feel in your body? ____

Worksheet: Three-Step Check-In Practice for Spotting Disguised Diet Culture

Message or trend I encountered:

____

1. Does it align with my values and intuition? ____

2. How does it make me feel—physically, emotionally, mentally?____

____

____

3. What is the honest impact if I follow it? ____

____

My inner skeptic says:

Worksheet: Compassionate Responses to Inner Food Police

Thought: ____

What is the deeper fear underneath it? ___________________________________

What is your lived experience that challenges this fear? _______________________

____

Compassionate response you'll offer instead:

"I hear you, but I choose to _________________________________**."**

Thought: ____

What is the deeper fear underneath it? ___________________________________

What is your lived experience that challenges this fear? _______________________

____

Compassionate response you'll offer instead:

"I hear you, but I choose to _________________________________**."**

Thought: ____

What is the deeper fear underneath it? _______________________________________

What is your lived experience that challenges this fear? _____________________________

____

Compassionate response you'll offer instead:

"I hear you, but I choose to _______________________________________**."**

Thought: ____

What is the deeper fear underneath it? _______________________________________

What is your lived experience that challenges this fear? _____________________________

____

Compassionate response you'll offer instead:

"I hear you, but I choose to _______________________________________**."**

Worksheet:
Advocating for Yourself with Nonviolent Communication

What situations make it hardest for you to speak up? Why?

What values are you protecting when you set a boundary?

What words help you stay rooted when you're feeling vulnerable?

Specific situation:____

Observation (without judgment): ____________________________________

____

Feeling: ____

Need: ____

Request:____

What value are you protecting by speaking up?

What support do you need to follow through?

Worksheet: Emotional Decoding Exercise

What just happened? (Describe the situation briefly):

What emotion do I think I'm feeling?

Can I allow this emotion to be here—just for now?

☐ Yes   ☐ Not yet   ☐ Maybe, with support

If I stay with it a little longer, does another emotion emerge?

What might I really need right now?

- ☐ Rest
- ☐ Connection
- ☐ Movement
- ☐ Reassurance
- ☐ Creative expression
- ☐ Boundaries
- ☐ Nourishment
- ☐ Other: _________

List three kind, feasible ways to meet this need:

1.

2.

3.

Worksheet:
Impermanence and Emotional Arcs

Everything you feel, think, or do is impermanent and follows a predictable arc: it arises, it peaks, and it dissolves. Use the prompts below to reflect on one **micro** arc and one **macro** arc from your own life.

Micro Arc (momentary experience)

What was the experience (e.g., craving, breath, meal, flash of emotion)?

What triggered its arising?

What did the peak feel like?

How did it eventually shift or dissolve?

What happened when you didn't interrupt the arc?

Macro Arc (longer-term experience)

What was the experience (e.g., grief, transition, chapter of life)?

When did it begin?

What have been its most intense moments?

Is it still unfolding, or has it resolved?

What has it taught you?

Zooming In and Zooming Out

Cultivating dual awareness can help you stay grounded while also holding a broader perspective.

Zoom In: What am I feeling in this moment—emotionally, physically, energetically?

Zoom Out: In the grander arc of this day, week, or season . . .what else is true?

Hold Both: What shifts when I let both realities be valid?

Worksheet: Emotional Eating Inventory

What do I tend to crave when I feel ...

Sad:

Anxious:

Lonely:

Overwhelmed:

In those moments, what does food offer me?
(Comfort? Numbing? Grounding? Familiarity?)

Does it help? Does it hurt? Does it depend?

Worksheet: Building Your Soothing Menu

Use this space to brainstorm other ways of caring for yourself when emotions run high. (These are *options,* not obligations. There is no moral hierarchy.)

Physical comfort:
(e.g., soft blanket, comfy clothes, stretching, warm bath)

Emotional connection:
(e.g., texting a friend, journaling, hugging a pet)

Sensory support:
(e.g., music, nature sounds, aromatherapy)

Expression or movement:
(e.g., drawing, dancing, pacing, singing)

Mind–body grounding:
(e.g., hand on heart, deep breathing, orienting to the room)

Worksheet: Exploring Your Other Hungers

I feel most alive when ...

I long for more ...

I wish someone would really see . . .

When I think of desire, I feel . . .

If I gave myself permission to want, I might discover . . .

Worksheet: Create a Personal Menu of Nourishment

Fill in the table below with your own examples of what feeds your emotional, physical, and spiritual well-being.

Nourishment Category	What You Crave	Examples or Ideas
Connection		
Creativity		
Movement		
Spirituality		
Pleasure		
Rest		
Play		
Purpose		
Beauty		

Which of these hungers have been going unmet?

How might tending to one of them soften the pressure you've placed on food?

Worksheet: Self-compassionate Statements

This formula can help you create supportive internal dialogue in moments of struggle:

1. When I feel . . .(name the emotion or situation)

2. I will remind myself . . .(compassionate truth)

3. And I will offer myself . . .(supportive action, perspective, or response)

Create your own three-part self-compassionate statement:

Use the prompts below to create your own self-compassionate statements based on situations in this chapter:

When I emotionally eat and feel regret, I will remind myself . . .

(e.g., I was coping in the only way I knew how in that moment.)

When I feel overwhelmed by emotion, I will offer myself . . .

(e.g., a deep breath, a hand on my heart, and the reminder that this too will pass.)

When I feel like I'm not making progress, I will remind myself . . .

(e.g., healing isn't a straight line, and showing up again is a sign of strength.)

Worksheet: Honoring What's Changing
(and how that could impact movement)

What has changed in my life or body recently that might affect how I move?

Am I allowing my movement practice to evolve—or trying to force it to stay the same?

What's something small I could try that fits my current needs?

Can I trust that changing my routine doesn't mean giving up—that it might be a deeper act of self-care?

Worksheet: Meal and Snack Builder

Combine carbs, proteins, fats, and fiber for more satisfaction and staying power.
Use the table below for ideas, and create your own!

Meal/Snack	Carb	Protein	Fat	Fiber	Notes on How It Felt
Example: *Breakfast bowl*	*Oats*	*Greek yogurt*	*Peanut butter*	*Berries*	*Kept me full until lunch, felt warm and comforting*

Worksheet: Nourishment Tracking

After meals or snacks, take a moment to notice:

- How is my energy? (sluggish, steady, jittery)
- How does my mood feel?
- Any digestive reactions?
- Did this meal satisfy me—emotionally or physically?

Meal/snack 1:

Meal/snack 2:

Meal/snack 3:

Meal/snack 4:

Meal/snack 5:

Meal/snack 6:

Worksheet: Adjusting Nutrition with Compassion

Take some time to reflect on what's changing—and how you might adapt with care.

What's shifted recently in my body, mind, or life?

What feelings come up around this change? Can I make space for them?

What kind of nourishment feels supportive now?

Is there anyone I can reach out to for support?

What gentle adjustment would help me feel more grounded?

Worksheet: Understanding My Fullness

What does fullness feel like in my body right now?

Are there early cues I've been missing?

What's my tendency—do I usually stop too early or go past my edge?

How does emotional context (stress, joy, loneliness) influence my experience of fullness?

How would I describe "enough" in my own words—not someone else's?

About the Author

Jenna Hollenstein is a nutrition therapist, author, and meditation teacher whose work explores food, embodiment, and meaning in a culture obsessed with control. She is the author of *Eat to Love* and the creator of the *Eat to Love Companion Workbook*, which invites readers to dismantle food rules without replacing them with subtler, more insidious ones.

Coming of age in the late twentieth century—amid diet culture, moral panic, and the promise that self-discipline would lead to safety—Jenna understands food struggles not as personal failures but as intelligent adaptations to their time. Her work draws from intuitive eating, trauma-informed mindfulness, Buddhist psychology, and feminist inquiry to examine how hunger is shaped, distorted, and reclaimed across a lifetime.

Rather than offering fixes or prescriptions, Jenna writes for readers who are tired of optimization and interested in truth: how bodies actually work, how culture gets under the skin, and what it means to live with agency and self-trust in midlife and beyond. She lives in New York with her family and continues to write about hunger in all its forms.

Also by Jenna Hollenstein

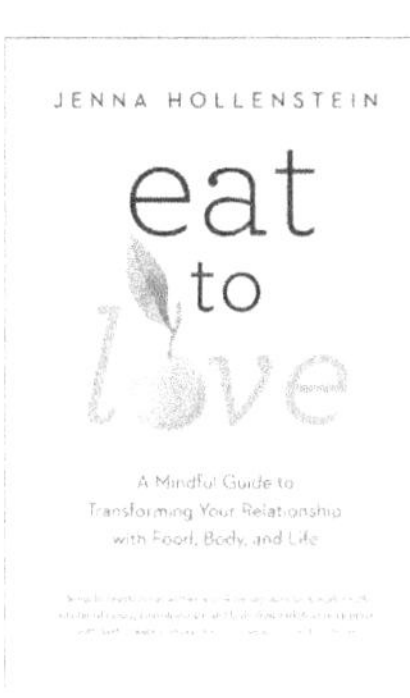

Eat to Love

A Mindful Guide to Transforming Your Relationship with Food, Body, and Life

January 2019

A Buddhist approach to conquering dieting insanity, which has insidiously infiltrated our culture and perpetuated an unnecessary source of suffering, especially for women. You don't need to be a Buddhist to use this book's practical tools to tap into your own internal wisdom.

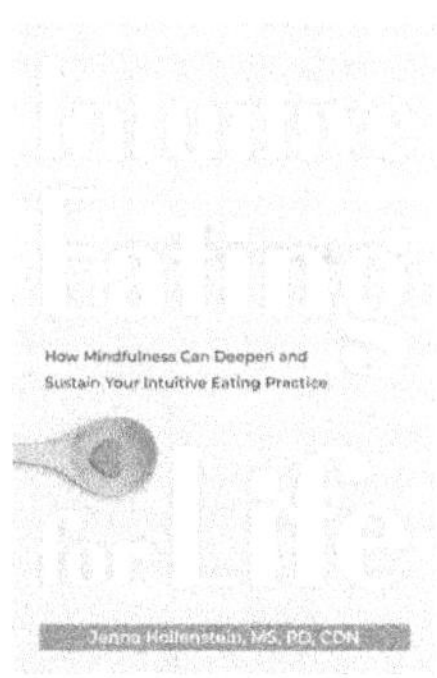

Intuitive Eating for Life

How Mindfulness Can Deepen and Sustain Your Intuitive Eating Practice

December 2022

Intuitive Eating is a powerful way to get off the diet roller coaster and take the guesswork out of mealtime. But if you're like many people, you may have trouble staying on track. Enter mindfulness! In this step-by-step guide, you'll learn to practice Intuitive Eating using the Four Foundations of Mindfulness, a classic Buddhist framework.

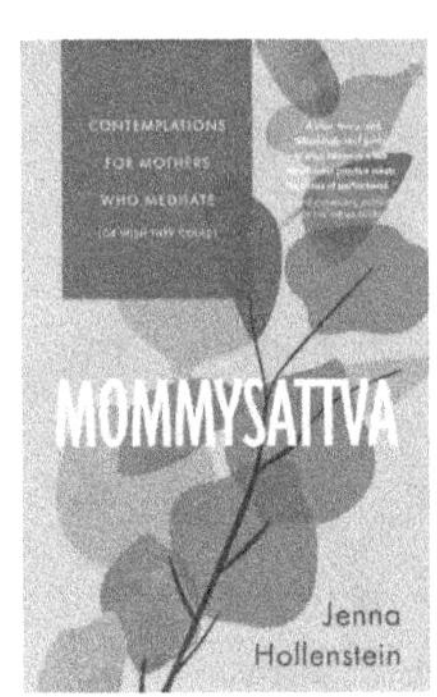

Mommysattva

*Contemplations for Mothers Who Meditate
(Or Wish They Could)*

September 2021

Mommysattva is a wise, funny, and refreshingly real guide to what happens when the ideals of mindfulness practice meet the chaos of everyday motherhood. Jenna Hollenstein writes from the heart of the parenting hurricane, offering ways to stay present, kind, and attuned to the mystery–even as the winds blow.

All available in paperback, ebook, and audiobook.